# NEUROLOGIC PEARLS

## ORRIN DEVINSKY, MD

Director, NYU–Mount Sinai Comprehensive Epilepsy Center
Director, Saint Barnabas Institute of Neurology and Neurosurgery
Professor of Neurology, Neurosurgery, and Psychiatry
New York University School of Medicine
New York, New York

## EDWARD FELDMANN, MD

Associate Professor
Department of Clinical Neurosciences
Brown University School of Medicine
Providence, Rhode Island

## HERMAN J. WEINREB, MD

Associate Professor of Clinical Neurology
New York University Medical Center
Chief, Division of Neurosciences
Hospital for Joint Diseases — Orthopaedic Institute
New York, New York

 F. A. DAVIS COMPANY • Philadelphia

F.A. Davis Company
1915 Arch Street
Philadelphia, PA 19103

Printed in Canada

Last digit indicates print number: 10 9 8 7 6 5 4 3 2 1

*Acquisitions Editor:* Robert W. Reinhardt
*Developmental Editor:* Bernice M. Wissler
*Production Editor:* Michael Schnee
*Cover Designer:* Louis J. Forgione

As new scientific information becomes available through basic and clinical research, recommended treatments and drug therapies undergo changes. The
authors and publisher have done everything possible to make this book accurate, up to date, and in accord with accepted standards at the time of publi-
cation. The authors, editors, and publisher are not responsible for errors or
omissions or for consequences from application of the book, and make no
warranty, expressed or implied, with regard to the contents of the book. Any
practice described in this book should be applied by the reader in accordance
with professional standards of care used with regard to the unique circumstances that may apply in each situation. The reader is advised always to check
product information (package inserts) for changes and new information regarding dose and contraindications before administering any drug. Caution
is especially urged when using new or infrequently ordered drugs.

**Library of Congress Cataloging-in-Publication Data**

Devinsky, Orrin.
    Neurologic pearls / Orrin Devinsky, Edward Feldmann, Herman J. Weinreb.
      p. ; cm.
    Includes bibliographical references and index.
    ISBN 0-8036-0433-5 (alk. paper)
    1. Nervous system—Diseases. 2. Neurology. I. Feldmann, Edward II.
Weinreb, Herman J., 1950-III. Title.
    [DNLM: 1. Nervous System Diseases—diagnosis. 2. Nervous System
Diseases—therapy. 3. Diagnostic Techniques, Neurological. 4. Nervous
System—physiopathology. WL 140 D495n 2000]
    RC346 .D48 2000
    616.8—dc21

                                        99-046439

# *Preface*

Neurologic illness presents challenging problems to the student of medicine as well as the practiced clinician. The brain, spinal cord, and peripheral nervous system have been studied extensively, yielding a vast, exponentially expanding amount of data. Yet their mysteries continue to outweigh our understanding.

Clinical neurology is a specialty that joins the science and the art of medicine. Patient history, anatomy and physiology, subtleties of examination, and the intellectual process of identifying the site and nature of the pathology form the essence of neurology. Our goal in this book is to provide students with a brief introductory overview of clinical neurology. We hope it will help them to understand the range of neurologic problems and thereby guide their diagnoses and treatment options.

The complexities of neuroanatomy and neurophysiology often limit a medical student's enthusiasm for clinical neurology. They should not. For clinical neurology, the patient is the textbook, not the basic science data. We hope this book will stimulate students' interest and understanding of an amazing and fascinating discipline. Neurology is a field in which our knowledge and therapeutic options are growing enormously, even while the number and complexity of unanswered questions never seems to diminish.

**OD**
**EF**
**HW**

# *Contents*

# *1*
### PART

# *Evaluating the Patient*

# 1

# Localization, History, and Exam

A patient's neurologic history focuses on the present illness and documents *common neurologic complaints*. The neurologic exam is directed by hypotheses generated from the history and identifies *neurologic signs*. The history and exam address three questions:

1. *Is neurologic disease present?* Neurologic disease is substantiated by **symptoms** (subjective reports from the patient, caregivers, or witnesses). The exam demonstrates **signs,** or objective findings that can be shown to observers. Lab tests (blood, neuroimaging, etc.) are thus signs. **PEARL: Non-neurologic conditions can mimic neural disease.** Syncope can mimic an epileptic seizure; claudication causes leg weakness; **conversion disorder** (the subconscious production of symptoms or signs that appear to be physical) and **malingering** (willful feigning) can mimic anything. **PEARL: Similarly, neurologic disorders can mimic or cause medical disorders.** For instance, subarachnoid hemorrhage can induce cardiac arrhythmias.

2. *Where is the lesion?* Clinical problem solving in neurology is unique. Whereas medicine focuses on the cause of the lesion, the primary task in neurologic diagnosis is *lesion localization.*
3. *What is the nature of the lesion?* Although it often helps to consider information on localization and pathophysiology simultaneously, keeping these diagnostic processes separate avoids contaminating one diagnostic process with errors made in the other.

## THE HISTORY

Accurate description of the present illness by the patient, supplemented by observers (relatives, friends, or witnesses, if available), is essential. Identify the *earliest* symptom of neurologic disease. Neurologic symptoms are often strange and difficult to describe. Make patients define terms such as dizziness or sciatica. Beware of attributing a bizarre complaint to hysteria.

**PEARL: There is no such thing as a "complete" neurologic examination: The clinician is directed by hypotheses generated from the history.** Appendix A lists components of a brief screening neurologic exam and the parts of the nervous system that are assessed.

### Common Neurologic Complaints

These are the common neurologic complaints:
- Headache and face pain
- Neck pain, back pain, shooting (radicular) pain
- Weakness (e.g., face, limbs, trunk, neck muscles)

- Sensory phenomena (e.g., numbness, burning, tingling in the face, limbs, or trunk)
- Voice, chewing, swallowing difficulties
- Muscle jerks, cramps, fasciculations
- Gait difficulties (e.g., falls, unsteadiness, ataxia, leg dragging)
- Dizziness and vertigo (subjective sense of movement)
- Hearing loss, tinnitus
- Visual disturbances (e.g., blurring, vision loss, diplopia, scotomata)
- Disordered thinking, attention, memory, behavior
- Language and communication disturbances
- Excessive daytime sleepiness, insomnia
- Sphincter disturbances (e.g., urinary or fecal incontinence, inability to void)
- Impaired libido, erectile or ejaculatory dysfunction
- Seizures, loss of consciousness, sudden behavioral changes

## Localization along the Neuraxis

The components of the neuraxis include:
- Central nervous system (CNS)
  - Cerebrum
  - White matter tracts
  - Basal ganglia
  - Cerebellum
  - Cranial nerves (CNs) I and II
  - Brainstem
  - Spinal cord
- Peripheral nervous system (PNS)
  - CNs III to XII
  - Roots
  - Spinal nerves
  - Cauda equina
  - Plexuses

- Peripheral nerves
- Neuromuscular junction
- Muscle
- Sensory receptors

The history and exam often point to a single localization along the neuraxis (see Appendix A). A single locus of neurologic dysfunction may not be found, however. Instead, the lesion may be multifocal (metastatic or demyelinating disease) or diffuse (toxic or metabolic).

**PEARL: The most common reasons for incorrect localization are incomplete knowledge of neuroanatomy and failure to elicit or identify clues from the history and exam.** Two other common localization errors are postulating *multifocal* disease when only one area is affected and placing the lesion too *centrally* (e.g., speech [but not language] problems may result from cranial nerve or muscle disorders as well as left frontal cortex lesions). Figures 1–1 and 1–2 show areas of the cerebral cortex that may be associated with motor and sensory problems.

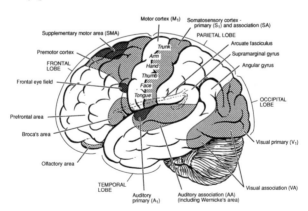

**Figure 1–1.** The cerebral cortex: lateral view. (From Devinsky O, Feldmann E, Weinreb HJ, and Wilterdink JL: The Resident's Neurology Book. Philadelphia, FA Davis, 1997, p 245, with permission.)

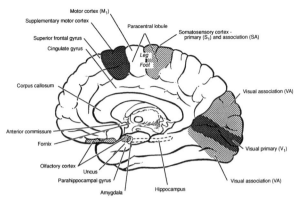

**Figure 1–2.** The cerebral cortex: medial view. (From Devinsky O, Feldmann E, Weinreb HJ, and Wilterdink JL: The Resident's Neurology Book. Philadelphia, FA Davis 1997, p 245, with permission.)

# THE NEUROLOGIC EXAMINATION

## General Observations

The mental status, CNs, motor, gait, and cerebellar exams are assessed partly by observing:

- Awareness, alertness, attitude, appropriate behavior, cooperation, eye contact
- Recitation of coherent history, richness of conversation, manner of speech
- Body posture, habitus, hygiene, general condition
- Spontaneous motor and verbal behaviors
- Emotional tone and affect: flat, labile, explosive, euphoric, depressed
- Coordinated motor acts (entering the room, fluidness and steadiness of gait, sitting, etc.)
- Eye movements; facial symmetry at rest, during speech, with emotion
- Involuntary movements, mannerisms, tics

# Mental Status Exam

## *General Mental Status*

The mental status exam begins with the sequential assessment of **arousal** (level of consciousness), orientation, attention, and comprehension. Impairments in these areas affect higher cognitive functions. **PEARL: When comprehension is impaired because of drowsiness or inattentiveness, functions such as memory, calculations, or *praxis* (the ability to plan and execute coordinated movements) cannot be accurately assessed.**

Many aspects of mental status may be observed:

- *Level of consciousness:* hyperalert, alert, somnolent, obtunded, stupor, coma. Describe specific behaviors (e.g., "Patient opened eyes only to painful stimulus, not voice") rather than just labels (e.g., "stupor"). When the patient is not alert and attentive, much of the mental status and sensory exams may be unobtainable or unreliable.
- *Orientation:* to time, place, examiner, situation.
- *Attention span:* digit span forward and backward.
- *Comprehension:* See later.
- *Behavior:* general appearance, interpersonal relations, motor and verbal spontaneity.
- *Mood and affect:* labile, apathetic, depressed, euphoric, irritable.
- *Disorders of thinking and perception:* circumstantiality, loose associations, paranoia, hallucinations, **illusions** (misperceptions of stimuli), **delusions** (false beliefs).

## *Specific Aspects of Mental Status*

**PEARL: In assessing mental functions, consider educational background, prior language skills, and cultural differences that may affect a patient's fund of knowledge.**

## Screening for Aphasia

To screen patients for **aphasia** (language disorder), assess their spontaneous speech, comprehension of spoken language, repetition of speech, naming, reading, and writing. Distinguish aphasia from confusion, **dysarthria** (difficulty with the mechanics of speech), and psychogenic disorders.

- *Spontaneous speech* can be assessed by considering:
  - Initiation
  - Sentence length
  - Fluency (nonfluent speech is slow, effortful, with frequent pauses)
  - **Prosody** (emotional inflection and melody of speech)
  - Articulation
  - Grammar
  - **Paraphasias** (abnormal words): **literal** (phonemic) paraphasias are replacements of letters or syllables, such as "slar" for "star"; **semantic** (verbal) paraphasias are word substitutions such as "lark" for "tomato" or creation of **neologisms** (new words)
  - Word-finding hesitations
  - **Circumlocutions** (talking around a word when unable to find it): "I had a burger, and also those greasy things that are long and thin, good with ketchup."
- *Comprehension* requires normal attention and can be assessed by simple and complex commands that do not require verbal output ("Point to the ceiling, and then touch your nose") and by yes or no questions ("Are you in a hotel? Do helicopters in South America eat their young?"). **PEARL: If comprehension is impaired, higher functions such as praxis and memory cannot be reliably assessed.**
- *Repetition* evaluates the ability to repeat single words, phrases, sentences, and syntacti-

cally complex phrases ("There are no ifs, ands, or buts about it." "The phantom soared across the foggy heath.").
- For *naming* ability, point to objects, parts of objects, colors, and body parts, and ask the patient to name them.
- For *reading* ability, ask the patient to read aloud and test comprehension.
- For *writing* ability, evaluate spontaneous writing (a spontaneous sentence) and writing to dictation (a paragraph about daily life).

## Assessing Memory

To assess *recent memory,* recite three words and ask the patient to repeat those words immediately (to make sure the patient was paying attention and heard you) and again at 5 minutes. Give both concrete (street name, color) and conceptual words ("honesty," "caring"); if impaired, test visual memory by pointing to three objects in the room.

To assess *remote memory,* ask about biographical and historic events (Kennedy assassination, Challenger explosion). The answers to questions about the person's own past must be confirmed by another source.

## Assessing Higher
## Cognitive Functions

If the patient demonstrates intact comprehension, other cognitive functions can be assessed:
- *Calculation and attention* (serial 7 subtractions from 100, months of the year backward).
- *General information* (recent presidents, current events).
- *Judgment, abstraction, and insight* (e.g., interpreting proverbs [watch for cultural bias]); similarities and differences (How are a cat and dog similar? Liberty and freedom?).
- *Writing and drawing* (test visuospatial and constructional abilities) (ask the patient to

draw a flower in a pot and a clock with hands, or to copy designs).

- **Apraxia** (inability to perform learned movements to command or imitation with intact comprehension, sensation, and strength). To test for apraxia, assign tasks of increasing difficulty. Ask the patient to respond to:
  - Midline commands (open eyes, stick out tongue)
  - Appendicular commands (pretend to salute the flag, comb hair, brush teeth, strike a match and light a cigarette)
  - Cross-midline commands (touch right thumb to left ear)
  - Two-step commands (touch left thumb to right cheek, then point to the ceiling)

### Testing for Agnosia

Presenting specific stimuli and testing recognition after demonstrating intact sensation can test for **agnosia** (impairments in comprehending or recognizing specific stimuli despite intact sensation). The varieties of agnosia are:

- **Auditory agnosia:** inability to recognize sounds and speech
- **Visual agnosia:** inability to recognize visual stimuli; **prosopagnosia** is the inability to identify faces
- **Astereognosia:** inability to identify objects placed in the palm, by touch
- **Anosognosia:** unawareness or denial of major neurologic deficits
- **Autotopagnosia:** inability to identify one's own limbs

## Cranial Nerve Testing

Assess CNs as well as supranuclear controls that influence the CNs. Attempt to determine whether the CN deficit is **supranuclear** (above the level of the brainstem CN nucleus), nuclear, or **infranuclear** (in the fibers from the nucleus to the periphery) (Fig. 1–3).

## *I: Olfactory Nerve*

Test each nostril with a nonastringent odor (e.g., coffee, cloves). Irritating odors (e.g., alcohol) stimulate CN V. If smell is impaired, examine the nasopharynx for blockage or discharge. Olfaction is tested when a head injury or frontal lobe tumor is suspected, or if the patient complains of loss of

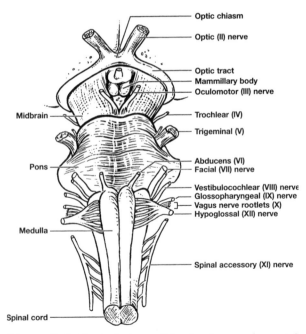

**Figure 1–3.** Ventral view of brain stem and cranial nerves. (From Devinsky O, Feldmann E, Weinreb HJ, and Wilterdink JL: The Resident's Neurology Book. Philadelphia, FA Davis, 1997, p 10, with permission.)

taste (often impaired because of loss of smell [anosmia]) or anorexia.

## II: Optic Nerve

Check visual acuity (corrected) in each eye. Acuity improved by looking through a pinhole suggests a refractive error, not a nerve lesion.

For the visual fields, test each eye separately and together by confrontation. Ask the patient to look at your nose when testing both eyes or to look at your open eye when testing each eye separately. A red hat pin is an ideal test object. Test each quadrant and check simultaneous stimulation of bilateral quadrants to detect **field neglect** (failure to detect a visual stimulus in part of the visual field only when there is a competing stimulus, not when that field is tested alone). Make sure the patient fixates on your eye. Screen by holding one or two fingers in each quadrant and ask the patient to sum them. **PEARL: Draw fields as seen by the patient in each eye.**

During the ophthalmoscopic exam, note the appearance of the disk, vessels, retina, and macula. Observe for pallor, swelling, nerve fiber layer loss, spontaneous venous pulsations, perivenous sheathing, arteriolar narrowing, AV nicking (localized constriction of retinal blood vessels), hemorrhages, and "cotton-wool spots."

A complete lesion of CN II causes monocular blindness. The lesion may be in the retina, disk (optic neuritis), or the optic nerve distal to the chiasm *(retrobulbar neuritis)*. Causes include neuritis (multiple sclerosis, inflammation), tumor, and trauma.

## Eye Movements and Pupils: Cranial Nerves III (Oculomotor), IV (Trochlear), VI (Abducens)

Check the position of the eyes in primary gaze and movements in the nine cardinal directions. Note whether the eyes move conjugately or

disconjugately. Does the patient complain of
**diplopia** (double vision)? For the pupils, note the
size, shape, reaction to direct and consensual
light, and **accommodation** (pupils constrict as
gaze is shifted from a far to a near point). Abnormally large pupils **(mydriasis)** and small pupils
**(meiosis)** result from many causes (Table 1–1).

### Table 1–1. PUPILLARY ABNORMALITIES

| Disorder | Causes | Notes |
|---|---|---|
| *Mydriasis (Large Pupil)* | | |
| Third nerve | Diabetes, aneurysm, trauma, temporal lobe herniation, tumor | Often acute. Diabetes: pupil usually spared |
| Tonic (Adie's pupil) | Idiopathic (viral?) | Often unilateral, ± arreflexia |
| Drug effects | Topical drugs | Scopolamine, atropine, cocaine |
| | Systemic drugs | Anticholinergics, antihistamines, MAO inhibitors, amphetamines |
| Iris | Surgery, trauma | |
| *Meiosis (Small Pupil)* | | |
| Horner's syndrome | Congenital, lesions of brainstem/cord, C8-T2 roots, Pancoast tumor, carotid, cavernous sinus, cluster headache | Ptosis, depression of upper lid, ± impaired ipsilateral upper facial sweating |
| Argyll-Robertson | Diabetes, syphilis | Irregular pupil |
| Pontine | Thrombosis, hemorrhage | Small, reactive pupil |
| Drug effects | Topical drugs | Glaucoma drugs |
| | Systemic drugs | Parasympathetic drugs (neostigmine), opioids |

MAO = monoamine oxidase.

Test for diplopia (use cross cover or red glass if necessary, as discussed later). Look for asymmetry of the corneal light reflex on primary gaze (Fig. 1–4). Determine the direction of image separation and direction of gaze in which separation is maximal and minimal. Check movements of each eye individually and maximally in all directions. Note **skew deviation** (one eye is higher than the other on the vertical axis; this implies brainstem or thalamic lesions).

For the cover-uncover **(cross cover)** test, as the patient looks at a target, one eye is covered and the examiner observes for movement in the uncovered eye. If there is no movement, the eye was looking at the target. If the eye moves to the nose, it was previously outwardly deviated, or **exotropic;** if the eye moves laterally, it was **esotropic.**

During the **red glass test** (looking at a white light with a red glass over one eye), the patient sees a red and white image. By covering each eye separately, one can determine which eye sees the "outer" (lateral) and which sees the "inner" image. The eye seeing the outer image usually has the weak extraocular muscle.

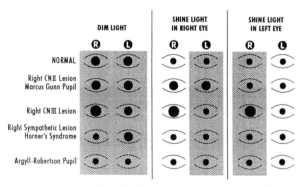

**Figure 1–4.** Pupillary light reactions. (From Józefowicz RF and Holloway RG, Case Studies in Neuroscience. Philadelphia, FA Davis, 1999, p 163, with permission.)

Check for **nystagmus** (rhythmic oscillations of the eyes, usually with a slow movement toward one side and a rapid corrective movement back). If it is present, record the direction and amplitude (fine, coarse) of the quick component, the plane of the nystagmus (is a rotational component present?), and the effects of different directions of gaze on the direction and amplitude of the nystagmus.

## III: Oculomotor Nerve

### Types of Disorders

**Ophthalmoparesis** (eye muscle weakness) affects medial, superior, and inferior recti and the inferior oblique muscles; **ophthalmoplegia** (paralysis of muscles supplied by CN III) abducts (unopposed lateral rectus) and depresses the eye (unopposed superior oblique). The eye is "down and out."

**Ptosis** (drooping of the upper eyelid) (Table 1–2) occurs because of levator palpebrae superioris weakness. It is best identified by comparing the space between the upper and lower lids and by noting the lid's relation to the limbus of the iris. Weakness of Müller's muscle, innervated by sympathetic fibers in both upper and lower eyelids, is seen in **Horner's syndrome** (small pupil without extraocular palsies). Both upper and lower lids are closer to the pupil. This syndrome is best identified in a dark room, which accentuates pupillary asymmetry and causes mild ptosis. **PEARL: Marked ptosis, with a large pupil or extraocular palsies, suggests a third nerve lesion.** Common causes of ptosis include third nerve palsies, myasthenia gravis, and Horner's syndrome.

Meiosis (pupillary constriction) comes from weakness of the pupillodilator muscle. An **Argyll-Robertson pupil** (the small, irregular pupil of neurosyphilis; see Fig. 1–4) is now usually due to diabetic autonomic neuropathy. Mydriasis (pupil-

**Table 1–2. PTOSIS AND PSEUDOPTOSIS**

| Disorder | Causes | Notes |
|---|---|---|
| Horner's syndrome | Lesions of sympathetic fibers (hypothalamus to cervical cord), C8-T2 roots to superior cervical ganglion, carotid sheath (cavernous sinus) | Weakness of Müller's muscle and meiosis; ± sweating over forehead; no extraocular palsy; best seen in dark room (pupillary asymmetry); upper and lower lids closer to the pupil |
| Third nerve | Diabetes, aneurysm, trauma, temporal lobe herniation, tumor | Often acute; often with extraocular palsy; best seen in bright room (pupillary asymmetry) |
| Myasthenia | Immune reaction to acetylcholine receptor | Often with extraocular palsy; increases with fatigue |
| Pseudoptosis | Lid tumors Hysterical Chronic Bell's palsy Enophthalmos Congenital | Neuromas, hemangiomas Check old photographs |
| | Lid laxity with aging Atopic conjunctivitis | |

lary dilatation) arises from weakness of the iris sphincter muscle. **Adie's pupil** (enlarged pupil from disorder of ciliary ganglion; 80% unilateral) usually occurs in young women and is benign. In both conditions, the pupil constricts with accommodation, not direct light.

*Loss of accommodation* comes from ciliary muscle weakness.

## Location and Causes of
## Third Nerve Lesions

To identify a brainstem lesion, look for contralateral limb weakness (corticospinal fibers), ataxia, tremor, and skew deviation. The causes may be vascular, multiple sclerosis, or glioma.

To identify a peripheral lesion, distinguish **compressive** lesions (parasympathetic fibers are peripheral and affected first, causing mydriasis and loss of light reflex before extraocular weakness) from **ischemic** lesions (medial fibers are affected first, causing ptosis and extraocular muscle weakness without mydriasis; vascular lesions are often "pupil sparing"). The causes of vascular lesions are usually idiopathic or microvascular (e.g., diabetes). The most common compressive lesions are aneurysms of the posterior communicating artery, tumors, and early temporal lobe herniation. Anticholinergics (topical or systemic) produce mydriasis without ophthalmoplegia. **PEARL: In comatose patients, third nerve lesions are usually *structural* when the pupil is involved and *metabolic* when the pupil is spared.**

## IV: Trochlear Nerve

Weakness of the superior oblique muscle results in vertical diplopia on downgaze and on looking away from the side of the lesion. The head may tilt to compensate, so the chin points to the side of the lesion. Isolated lesions are rare. Trauma is the most common cause; vascular disease and dorsal brainstem tumors are other possibilities.

## VI: Abducens Nerve

These lesions weaken the lateral rectus muscle and result in medial deviation, impaired abduction, and horizontal diplopia. To identify a brainstem locus, look for ipsilateral facial weakness and numbness and contralateral limb weakness. Causes may be vascular or tumor. Peripheral involvement of CN VI occurs with lesions at the tip of the petrous bone, cavernous sinus, or orbit. In meningeal disease, vascular insults, tumors, or trauma, increased intracranial pressure may stretch CN VI and cause a *false localizing sign.* (The lesion may be remote from the sixth nerve.)

### V: Trigeminal Nerve

Assess sensation (tactile, temperature, pain) in the three territories of CN V on the face. **PEARL: Deficits from pure trigeminal lesions do not extend onto the pinna or beyond the angle of the mandible.** If a deficit is reported, test sensation inside the mouth and on the tongue. Pain may occur. Persistent sensory loss or motor deficit is atypical in trigeminal neuralgia (*tic douloureux*).

Feel the temporalis and masseter bulk when the patient is chewing (note ipsilateral atrophy, weakness on jaw closure). Note the direction of the jaw opening ( jaw deviates to the side of the lesion due to weak lateral pterygoids) and the patient's ability to move the jaw laterally against resistance.

To test the *corneal reflex,* apply cotton gently from sclera to cornea and see that both eyes blink. The afferent limb is carried in CN $V_1$ (the first division of CN V) and the efferent limb by CN VII.

The *jaw jerk reflex* is tested by placing a finger over the patient's chin with the mouth partially open and relaxed; tap the finger gently with a reflex hammer and observe for unequivocally brisk jaw contraction. The sensory and motor limbs are carried by CN $V_3$. This reflex is exaggerated in bilateral supranuclear lesions, such as bilateral subcortical infarcts or motor neuron disease.

### VII: Facial Nerve

Note the degree and distribution of facial muscle involvement and the symmetry of the facial (nasolabial) folds during different movements: voluntary ("Show me your teeth."), conversation, and spontaneous emotions (e.g., smiling). Other facial muscles innervated by CN VII include the frontalis (wrinkling the forehead), orbicularis oculi (closing the eyes) and buccinator (producing pronounced labials, such as "paper bag").

Facial muscle weakness may result from different lesion sites. A *peripheral lesion* affects the entire face; if taste on the anterior two-thirds of the tongue is affected, the lesion is proximal to the stylomastoid foramen, where the chorda tympani joins the facial nerve in the middle ear. Weakness of the frontalis is present. Causes may be idiopathic (Bell's palsy), sarcoidosis, meningitis, trauma, Lyme disease, diabetes, acoustic neuroma, and herpes oticus (Ramsay Hunt syndrome—check for vesicles in the external auditory canal).

A *brainstem (nuclear) site* affects the entire face plus the **lateral rectus** (sixth nerve fiber in the brainstem); there may be other CN or brainstem findings. Causes include stroke, multiple sclerosis, and glioma. Supranuclear facial palsy affects lower facial muscles, and may be limited to voluntary ("Show me your teeth.") or **mimetic** (emotional expression) acts. Causes include stroke, tumor, trauma, and multiple sclerosis.

Taste and lacrimation are not routinely tested, but these tests should be included when peripheral CN VII problems are suspected. To test taste, paint the lateral two-thirds of the protruded tongue on each side with a cotton swab soaked in sugar water; then have the patient raise a hand (without retracting his tongue) if taste is perceived. To test lacrimation (Schirmer's test), suspend a strip of litmus or filter paper from each lower eyelid and observe the amount of accumulated moisture (less than 5 mm is abnormal).

## VIII: Acoustic Nerve

To test the cochlear division, begin with an otoscopic exam. Note the patient's understanding of normal speech, ability to hear a tuning fork (512 Hz preferred) that is perceptible to an examiner with normal hearing, or whether the patient can hear the examiner's fingers being rubbed together with opposite ear occluded. Whisper "22" and "44" in each ear with the opposite ear occluded. Hearing impairment may be due to conductive or sensorineural deficits.

For **Weber's test,** a tuning fork (512 Hz preferred) is placed over the teeth, forehead, or vertex. Sound is normally symmetrical. If an ear is occluded because of conductive impairment, sound is heard louder on that side. With sensorineural deafness, sound is less on the involved side. **Rinne's test** compares bone and air conduction. A tuning fork (512 Hz preferred) is placed firmly against the mastoid until sound is no longer heard; then it is moved next to the external auditory meatus, where sound should still be heard. With conductive deafness, the sound will not be heard.

To test the vestibular division, determine whether nystagmus is present. Nystagmus results from labyrinthine, brainstem, and cerebellar lesions.

Other vestibular tests include:
- Effect of changing eye position on nystagmus.
- Vertigo induced by rapid head nodding while staring at the examiner's eyes.
- Unsteadiness in walking or standing, with eyes open and closed.
- *Past pointing:* After first touching the examiner's finger, the patient closes his or her eyes and raises the fully extended arm to return to the examiner's finger (movement occurs at shoulder).
- *Caloric testing* (oculovestibular reflex): See Chapter 17 regarding the procedure for pa-

tients in coma. In awake subjects, however, 10 to 20 mL of tepid water (which is cool relative to the body) is effective and much better tolerated than the ice water used in comatose patients. With tepid water in awake subjects, the fast component of nystagmus is opposite the stimulated ear (use the mnemonic "COWS": cold-opposite; warm-same).

- Oculocephalic (doll's eyes) reflex (see Chapter 17).
- *Nylen-Barány maneuver:* The patient sits on the end of the examination table and is placed abruptly in a lying position, with the head hanging down 45° and inclined toward the ground. **Positional vertigo** (perception of rotation or movement of subject or environment) and nystagmus may be elicited. With repeated maneuvers, note the latency, duration, and fatigability of evoked nystagmus.

Lesions of CN VIII result from involvement of:

- *End organs (cochlea or labyrinth):* Causes may be viral, **Ménière's disease** (abrupt attacks of vertigo accompanied by tinnitus, deafness, and a pressure sensation in ear, usually unilateral), trauma, or drugs (aminoglycosides).
- *Nerve:* The cause may be trauma or an acoustic neuroma.
- *Brainstem:* On entering the brainstem, auditory pathways become bilaterally crossed; unilateral hearing loss is quite rare with intra-axial lesions.
- *Lesions of vestibular nuclei or pathways (from stroke, multiple sclerosis, glioma):* These lesions cause nystagmus and vertigo.

### *IX and X: Glossopharyngeal and Vagus Nerves*

These CNs are clinically inseparable. Visceral functions of CN X are evaluated by observing pulse, respiration, and oculocardiac and carotid sinus reflexes.

*Supranuclear* lesions affecting motor functions of CNs IX and X are clinically evident only if bilateral; unilateral nuclear or infranuclear lesions may also produce symptoms. Note symmetrical elevation of the soft palate on phonation or gagging (motor limb of gag reflex). The uvula deviates away from the side of the lesion. **PEARL: Evaluate swallowing by watching the patient drink water. Indirect laryngoscopy assesses vocal cord function.**

Abnormalities produce nasal speech, hoarseness, inability to articulate "ga, ga, ga" or "ka, ka, ka," and diminished speech amplitude. Nasal regurgitation of swallowed liquids or an inability to maintain puffed cheeks unless the nose is occluded indicates palatal weakness.

Sensation is assessed by gently stimulating the left and right sides of the posterior pharynx and soft palate with a cotton swab and noting the quality and symmetry of the gag reflex (sensory limb). Absence of the gag reflex (from lower motor neuron [LMN] lesions) or marked hyperactivity of the gag reflex (from upper motor neuron [UMN] lesions) is clinically significant.

## XI: Spinal Accessory Nerve

Assess the strength and bulk of the sternocleidomastoid (lateral neck rotation) and upper trapezius (shoulder shrug) muscles. Infranuclear (peripheral) lesions usually affect these muscles.

## XII: Hypoglossal Nerve

With LMN lesions, atrophy and fasciculations are seen in the resting tongue. Assess deviation of the tongue when protruded. Asymmetry caused by facial weakness may be confusing. Therefore, compare the median raphe of the tongue to a line from the point of the nose to the point of the chin. With an LMN lesion, the tongue deviates to the side of the lesion. In acute UMN lesions, the tongue deviates to the other side.

Check rapidly repeated lingual pronunciation: "newly laid linoleum," "lollipop," "la, la." These are often impaired in bilateral supranuclear lesions.

## Motor System and Coordination

This section includes pyramidal, extrapyramidal, LMN, and cerebellar functions and is organized by exam performance, not neurologic system (Appendix B).

### *General Observations*

Observe the natural gait and the way the patient walks on heels, toes, and in tandem (these latter movements are heavily dependent on cerebellar pathways). Note slowness and difficulty initiating or completing movements (often an extrapyramidal sign). **PEARL: With extrapyramidal or UMN lesions, automatic arm swing when walking is decreased.** Note circumduction of the leg (rotated in a semicircle, often with flexed, adducted arm with an UMN lesion). **PEARL: Hopping on each leg is a sensitive screen for pyramidal and sensory impairment.**

Study station and posture with the patient's eyes open and closed. Evaluate arm and leg extension with the patient's eyes closed, noting up or down drift. With UMN lesions, the arm drifts down with pronation of the hand and flexion of the arm; there may be hypertonia. In cerebellar lesions, the arm drifts down without pronation of the hand and passive limb tone may be hypotonic. With sensory loss, the arm drifts up from lack of proprioceptive input; there may also be slow finger movements (pseudoathetosis). Note any abnormal movements, such as tremor, dyskinesia, chorea, and athetosis. Depress each limb with a vigorous tap, and note excessive resistance (UMN or extrapyramidal) or excessive rebound (cerebellar). To assess proprioception in the upper limbs, have the patient touch the tip of the nose with arms extended and eyes closed ("Romberg of upper limbs").

Assess rapid movements. With diadochokinesis, the patient pronates and supinates one hand in the palm of the other rapidly. Clumsiness or failure reflects cerebellar more than corticospinal impairment. Check the dexterity of finger and toe movements (corticospinal function) by having patients rapidly tap each finger, wiggle their toes, and rapidly tap the sole with the heel planted.

Assess coordination by performing the **finger-nose-finger test,** in which the patient alternately touches the nose and the examiner's finger, which moves randomly from spot to spot, and the **heel-shin test,** in which the patient places one heel on the opposite tibia (shin) and runs the heel smoothly down the shin to the ankle. Have the patient rapidly stomp each heel while seated. Note any dysmetria, past pointing, and intention tremor.

Note micrographia (seen in parkinsonism) and tremor in handwriting. Note dysarthria, scanning, and staccato and explosive speech. Are there spontaneous involuntary movements? In the case of tremor, note the amplitude and rate and whether maximal with rest, sustained posture, or movement.

### *Specific Muscle Survey*

Inspect for muscle contour, bulk, atrophy (compare to opposite side; dominant arm is often mildly larger), and fasciculation. **PEARL: Severe muscle atrophy usually denotes an LMN lesion.**

Note resting posture (e.g., external rotation of a lower extremity while supine occurs in pyramidal weakness and hip fracture).

Evaluate muscle tone in all limbs and in the neck:

- **Flaccid:** absence of tone; muscle is moved without any resistance.
- **Spastic:** muscle tension increases during passive stretch, from exaggerated muscle stretch reflex. With increased velocity of stretch, resistance is increased. In corticospinal tract lesions, sudden stretch initially increases resistance, followed quickly by "give-way" relaxation (*clasp-knife*).
- **Spasm:** sustained muscle contraction. **PEARL: In spasticity, the limb can be fully extended with steady, gentle traction. In *fibrotic contracture,* the limb cannot be extended owing to fixed soft-tissue changes.**
- **Dystonia:** sustained abnormal posture of trunk or limbs, caused by cocontraction of agonists and antagonists. It is usually due to basal ganglia lesions or adverse drug effects (neuroleptics, levodopa).
- **Hypotonia** is associated with acute corticospinal lesions. Chronic hypotonia implicates cerebellar or LMN injury.
- **Cogwheel rigidity** (lead-pipe stiffness, often with superimposed "ratchet tremor") occurs in extrapyramidal lesions.
- **Paratonia ("*gegenhalten*"):** dynamic resistance to passive movements that increases in proportion to the examiner's effort to change limb position. It occurs in metabolic encephalopathies, extrapyramidal lesions, and diffuse cerebral dysfunction (advanced dementia).
- **Myotonia:** sustained muscle contraction, with slowed muscle relaxation after active movement (the "never-ending handshake"). It is a hallmark of myotonic dystrophies.

### *Testing Muscle Strength*

Muscle strength is graded on a scale like that shown in Table 1–3. Consider the effects of gravity. Do not be misled by pain restricting movement, contractures limiting range of motion, ligament or tendon injuries, or trick movements (e.g., other synergists, which are muscles that assist in a given movement). **PEARL: Identify give-way weakness: If the patient can briefly exert maximal strength, but then suddenly loses strength, a functional disorder may be present.**

Weakness of particular muscles suggests a lesion at or above the vertebral segments listed in Table 1–4.

## Sensory System

When numbness or sensory loss is reported, map the involved area with a cotton swab stick and pin. With equivocal findings, repeat the exam later. Distinguish peripheral (nerve, root, dermatome [Fig. 1–5]) lesions from central (cord and brainstem white matter tracts, thalamus, internal capsule, sensory cortex) lesions.

In testing light touch or pain, move from areas of lesser to those of greater sensation. Intermittently

### Table 1–3. GRADING OF MUSCLE STRENGTH*

0 No contraction of muscle
1 Muscle contraction, no movement
2 Movement with gravity eliminated
3 Movement against gravity
4 Movement against moderate resistance
5 Full power

*Plus (+) or minus (−) may be added to muscle strength in the 3 to 5 range (e.g., 3+, 5−) to quantify subtle weakness.

## Table 1–4. SEGMENTAL INNERVATION OF MUSCLES

| Region | Muscles | Segmental Innervation* |
|---|---|---|
| Neck | Trapezius | C2-C4 |
| | Sternocleidomastoid | C1-C3 |
| | Diaphragm | C4 |
| Shoulder/ upper chest | Deltoid | **C5,** C6 |
| | Supraspinatus, infraspinatus | **C5,** C6 |
| | Pectoralis major | C5-C8, T1 |
| Arm | Biceps, brachialis anterior, brachioradialis | C5, C6 |
| | Triceps | C6-C8 |
| Forearm | Wrist extensors | C6-C8 |
| | Extensors of MP joints | C6-C8 |
| | Wrist flexors | C7, C8, T1 |
| | Radial deviation of wrist | C6, C7 |
| | Ulnar deviation of wrist | C7, **C8,** T1 |
| | Supination | C5, C6 |
| | Pronation | C6-C8 |
| Hand | Lumbricals, interossei, opposition of thumb | C8, **T1** |
| | Abductor, flexor pollicis brevis | C7, **C8** |
| Pelvic girdle | Iliopsoas | Tl2, **L1, L2,** L3 |
| | Glutei | **L4, L5,** S1 |
| Thigh | Quadriceps | L2-L4 |
| | Abductors | L2-L5, S1 |
| | Adductors | **L2, L3,** L4 |
| | Semitendinosus, semimembranosus | L5, **S1,** S2, |
| | Biceps femoris | L5, **S1,** S2 |
| Leg | Gastrocnemius and soleus | S1, S2 |
| | Tibialis anterior | **L4,** L5 |
| | Peronei | L5, S1 |
| Foot | Short plantar muscles | S1, S2 |
| Anus† | External sphincter | S2, S3, S4 |
| Bladder | (Smooth muscle) | S2, S3 |

*Boldface type signifies predominant innervation.
†Rectal exam is part of the motor exam to determine external sphincter tone (and palpate for masses).

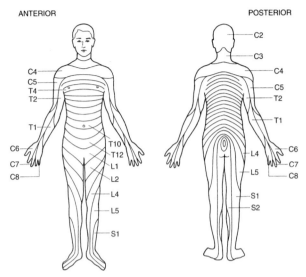

**Figure 1–5.** The sensory dermatomes. (From Nolan MF: Introduction to the Neurologic Examination. Philadelphia, FA Davis, 1996, p 167, with permission.)

ask the patient to point to the area stimulated **(topognosia).** Use a sterile pin to test pain, alternating sharp and dull stimuli, and ask for a rapid response. A cotton swab stick to test light touch may uncover an area of sensory loss better than pinprick. Testing temperature (warm or cool stimuli) produces results often more reliable than pain sensation (they use the same pathway). Always test temperature sensation if altered pain or touch sensation suggests a dermatomal lesion or a spinal cord intramedullary process (syrinx, tumor).

**Paresthesias** (tactile hallucinations) and **dysesthesias** (unpleasant, distorted tactile sensations) result from abnormal exteroception (peripheral or central nervous system).

Sensation from deep tissues (muscles, ligaments, bones, tendons, and joints) is tested with:

- *Vibration:* Using a 128- or 256-Hz tuning fork, test threshold by firmly tapping fork and asking the patient to report the cessation of vibration (compare with your own limbs).
- *Position and movement sensation (proprioception):* Move distal joints (ensure that patient cannot see movement); also move a limb into a certain posture with patient's eyes closed and then ask patient to describe or to imitate posture with the other limb. Begin with the toes or distal interphalangeal joints; if joint movement perception is impaired, advance to more proximal joints (ankle, wrist).
- *Deep pain:* Loss of pain suggests a complete nerve lesion.
- *Romberg maneuver:* Steadiness is observed while the patient stands with the feet together and the eyes open, then closed. **PEARL: Marked unsteadiness and falling with eyes closed suggests defective position sensation (posterior columns); marked unsteadiness with eyes open suggests a cerebellar lesion.**

After determining that primary sensation is intact, test cortical (parietal) sensation:

- **Stereognosis**—the ability to identify shapes and sizes by touch with preserved exteroceptive and proprioceptive sensation (light touch, pinprick, joint position, and vibration).
- **Palm writing** (*graphesthesia*): With the patient's eyes closed, have the patient report numbers drawn in each palm.
- *Two-point discrimination:* Normal values (mm) to detect two separate tactile stimuli: fingertip (2.5), dorsum of hand (25), dorsum of feet (35), back (45).
- *Double simultaneous stimulation (DSS):* loss often occurs in association with left-sided neglect following a right parietal lesion. Stimu-

lation of symmetrical body parts (e.g., both hands) is more reliable but less sensitive than asymmetrical parts (hand and opposite cheek).

• *Localization of sensation (topognosia):* Impairment suggests a contralateral parietal lesion.

## Reflexes

The muscle should be in a state of slight contraction. The force of the stimulus should be just above threshold. Start gently (i.e., light taps). If lower limb reflexes are absent, patients should pull their clenched hands apart and clench their teeth. These reinforcement maneuvers may cause absent knee and ankle jerks to appear.

Rate reflexes by this scale:

0 absent despite reinforcement
1 sluggish, hypoactive
2 active
3 very lively, could be normal or mildly pathologically hyperactive
4 transient clonus, pathologically brisk
5 sustained clonus

Table 1–5 summarizes the examination and localization of deep tendon reflexes, and Table 1–6, superficial cutaneous reflexes.

Certain reflexes signify diffuse cerebral or frontal dysfunction: snout, suck, grasp, rooting, and **palmomental** (mentalis contraction with light stroking of the ipsilateral thenar region). Some normal young adults and cognitively healthy older persons exhibit palmomental or snout responses. Involuntary eye closure with repeated glabellar tapping **(Meyerson's sign)** is frequent in Parkinson's disease and in diffuse cerebral dysfunction.

**Table 1-5. DEEP TENDON REFLEXES**

| Reflex | Exam | Effect | Localization |
|---|---|---|---|
| Jaw jerk | Tap center of slightly opened lower jaw. | Brisk jaw closure | CN V |
| Orbicularis oculi* | Fold skin over temple between fingers; strike finger. | Contraction of both orbicularis oculi muscles | CN VII |
| Sternocleidomastoid | Tap muscle at clavicular origin. | Muscle contraction | C3-4 |
| Pectoral | Arm abducted, tap finger over tendon to humerus. | Adduction, internal rotation of arm | C5-T1 (lateral pectoral nerve) |
| Biceps | Tap thumb placed over biceps tendon. | Elbow flexion | C5-6 (musculo-cutaneous nerve) |
| Brachioradialis | With forearm semipronated, tap styloid process of radius. | Elbow flexion | C5-6 (radial nerve) |
| Pronator | Tap palmar forearm medial to styloid process of radius. | Forearm pronation | C6 (median nerve) |
| Triceps | Tap just above olecranon. | Elbow extension | C6-7 (radial nerve) |
| Finger flexion | Tap ends of semiflexed fingers. | Finger flexion | C6-T1 (medial and ulnar) |
| Adductor | Tap medial condyle of femur. | Leg adduction | L2-4 (obturator nerve) |
| Patellar | Tap patellar tendon. | Knee extension | L2-4 (femoral nerve) |
| Tibialis posterior | Tap above and behind medial malleolus. | Foot inversion | L5-S1 (tibial nerve) |
| Biceps femoris | Tap head of fibula. | Posterior upper leg contraction | L5-S2 (sciatic nerve) |
| Achilles | Tap Achilles tendon. | Foot plantar flexion | S1-1 (tibial nerve) |

*A reflex, but not from deep tendon.

## Table 1–6. THE SUPERFICIAL CUTANEOUS REFLEXES

| Reflex | Exam | Effect | Localization |
|--------|------|--------|--------------|
| Corneal | Touch corneoscleral junction. | Bilateral eyelid closure | CNs V and VII |
| Palatal/ pharyngeal | Touch soft palate and pharynx. | Palate elevation and gagging | CNs IX and X |
| Palmar | Stroke palmar surface of hand. | Finger flexion | C8-T1 |
| Abdominal | Stroke skin of abdomen: Upper Middle Lower | Abdominal wall contraction | Upper T7-9 Middle T9-11 Lower T11-L1 |
| Cremasteric | Stroke medial upper thigh. | Scrotal and testicular elevation | L1-2 |
| Gluteal | Stroke skin of buttocks. | Gluteal contraction | L4-S1 |
| Bulbocavernosus | Place pressure on glans penis. | Contraction of bulbocavernosus | S3-4 |
| Anal wink | Stroke perianal region. | Contraction of external anal sphincter | S2-4 |
| Babinski's* | Stroke lateral sole of foot. | Dorsiflexion of great toe, fanning of other toes | Pyramidal tract lesion above L4 |

*Absent in normal individuals.

## Autonomic Exam

When autonomic dysfunction is suspected, **orthostatic vital signs** (blood pressure and pulse after lying, sitting, and standing for at least 2 minutes) should be recorded. Piloerection, dermatographia, carotid sinus, oculocardiac, sinus arrhythmia, and sweating (tested with iodine-cornstarch) are other autonomic reflexes that can be tested at the bedside.

## Other Components of the Neurologic Exam

- *Muscle percussion (not reflexes):* myotonia, myotatic irritability, myokymia, fasciculation
- Meningeal and root *stretch maneuvers:*
  - Voluntary and passive neck flexion.
  - **Kernig sign:** While flexing the thigh of a recumbent patient to 90°, attempted extension of the leg at knee is painful and limited by reflex spasm.
  - **Brudzinski's sign:** Rapid passive flexion of the head while supine elicits reflex flexion of thighs and legs.
  - **Patrick's test (FABERE—Flexion, ABduction, External Rotation, and Extension):** Evoked pain reproducing the patient's back pain complaint implicates sacroiliac or hip joint disease.
- *Cranium:* size, shape, palpation, bruits
- *Spine:*
  - Percussion tenderness, facet joint tenderness, lordosis, kyphosis, scoliosis, auscultation (dural AV malformation)
  - *Cervical spine:* Range of motion in extension, flexion, lateral bending, and rotation; paravertebral spasm
  - *Lumbar spine:* Range of motion in extension, flexion, lateral bending (thoracic spine), and rotation (thoracic spine); paravertebral spasm.
  - *Straight-leg raising:* While the patient lies supine, pain and limited movement during

leg elevation with the knee extended and prompt relief by knee flexion suggests irritation of the sciatic nerve or its roots **(Laségue's sign). PEARL: In disk herniation, straight-leg raising of the opposite leg may evoke radicular pain on the affected side.**

- *Reverse straight-leg raising:* While the patient lies prone, pain and limited movement during straight leg elevation suggest that the femoral nerve or upper lumbar roots are being irritated.
- *Palpation:*
  - *Peripheral nerves:* ulnar, peroneal, sciatic, greater occipital; **Tinel's sign** (induced by percussion of the median nerve at carpal tunnel)
  - *Muscles:* tenderness and consistency
  - *Arteries:* carotid, temporal, radial, facial
- *Auscultation:* cranial, orbital, carotid, vertebral bruit

## DRAWING CONCLUSIONS

The common neurologic complaints from the history and the signs on exam are integrated to determine whether neurologic disease is present and, if so, at what locations. Before invoking multiple or diffuse lesions, attempt to identify a single locus in the neuraxis that explains all the symptoms and signs. Reexamination clarifies uncertain findings and identifies progression or improvement of a disorder. After the localization and diagnosis are made, integrate new information from further history and lab testing, then reconsider your conclusions. Even experts are often wrong!

# 2

# *Diagnostic Studies*

## LUMBAR PUNCTURE

Lumbar puncture (LP) is commonly performed in the emergency room, on the inpatient service, or in outpatient areas. It is used to diagnose meningitis, encephalitis, sarcoidosis, subarachnoid hemorrhage, leakage of blood into the subarachnoid space from intracerebral hemorrhage, and meningeal carcinomatosis. To identify cancer cells in a patient with suspected meningeal carcinomatosis, multiple LPs may be needed for cytology exams. LP measures elevated or low intracranial pressure. Besides its diagnostic uses, LP allows administration of intrathecal antibiotic therapy or chemotherapy for meningeal carcinomatosis.

The results of cerebrospinal fluid (CSF) culture are valid even when fluid is obtained up to 4 hours after antibiotics are administered. However, if antibiotics are administered while the computed tomography (CT) scan is performed to rule out a mass lesion and if LP is delayed for more than 4 hours, bacterial antigens can be detected in the CSF. The markers are identified via agglutination tests for *Neisseria meningitidis,*

*Haemophilus influenzae,* and *Streptococcus pneumoniae.*

Prior to LP, prothrombin time, partial thromboplastin time, and platelet count should be checked.

**PEARL: Do not perform LP if the skin overlying the puncture site is infected or the underlying tissues are likely to be infected. If a patient has papilledema or focal neurologic signs, obtain a CT scan of the brain first. If CT confirms a mass lesion with herniation, shift of tissue, or obliteration of CSF pathways, do *not* perform LP unless active infection is strongly suspected and measures to reduce intracranial pressure have been instituted.**

LP should be performed or supervised by an experienced physician. Place the patient in the left lateral decubitus position. Before LP, the skin should be made aseptic with serial iodine and alcohol washes. Sterile gloves and drapes should be used. All the equipment including the manometer should be ready before the puncture. Palpate the L3-4 interspace of the spinous processes at the level of the superior iliac crest (Fig. 2–1). The skin should be anesthetized with lidocaine. The legs should be relaxed until immediately before the puncture, at which time the legs are flexed into the abdominal area. Pass a #20 gauge spinal needle through the skin and deeper tissues toward the subarachnoid space. Use a #22 gauge needle if the patient has borderline coagulability, such as a low platelet count. A longer needle is needed for obese patients.

The bevel of the needle should be parallel to the long axis of the spine, with the needle placed parallel to the examination table and tilted superiorly toward the umbilicus. After a firm pop is felt as the needle pierces the dura, remove the stylet and check the spinal needle after every 2 mm of advancement for the appearance of CSF. Do not advance the needle until after the stylet is replaced.

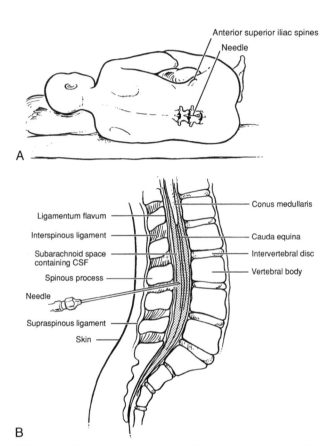

**Figure 2–1.** Lumbar puncture (*A*) Patient position. (*B*) Needle placement, showing course through the skin and ligaments to reach the sac containing cerebrospinal fluid. A "pop" is often felt as the needle passes through the ligamentum flavum. (Adapted from Devinsky O, Feldmann E, Weinreb HJ, and Wilterdink JL: The Resident's Neurology Book. Philadelphia, FA Davis, 1997, pp 28, 29, with permission.)

When CSF appears, the needle should be rotated 90° with the open end of the bevel facing the patient's head, and the fluid collected. Before collecting fluid, measure the opening pressure with the patient prone with legs extended and relaxed. LP can also be performed with the patient sitting, in which case the pressure can be adjusted for the change in column height, or the patient can lie down. Measure the closing pressure after fluid is removed. Suggested tests for routine spinal fluid evaluation are listed in Table 2–1.

If the patient has raised intracranial pressure, neurologic vital signs (e.g., level of consciousness, pupil size, and light reflex) should be observed every 15 minutes for several hours after the procedure. If signs of herniation, such as diminished consciousness and pupillary enlargement, develop during the procedure, replace the stylet to minimize the drainage of fluid, and emergently evaluate and treat the patient.

**PEARL: If the spinal needle advances too far, trauma to veins anterior to the dura causes bloody CSF (traumatic tap). If the bloody fluid is immediately spun down, traumatic tap can be differentiated from subarachnoid hemorrhage.** The supernatant can be tested by dipstick for bilirubin; presence of

**Table 2–1. TESTING SUGGESTIONS FOR CEREBROSPINAL FLUID OBTAINED BY LUMBAR PUNCTURE**

| | |
|---|---|
| Tube 1 | Protein and glucose |
| Tube 2 | Gram stain and culture |
| Tube 3 | Cell count and differential |
| Tube 4 | Cytologic testing<br>Staining for acid-fast bacilli<br>Cryptococcal antigen<br>Serologic testing for syphilis and Lyme disease<br>Viral titers<br>Immunoglobulin profiles<br>Oligoclonal banding |

bilirubin by dipstick suggests that blood has been present in the fluid for at least several hours and confirms the diagnosis of subarachnoid hemorrhage rather than traumatic tap. The supernatant should be sent to the lab for colorimetric testing for xanthochromia, which also suggests that blood has been present for hours, supporting a diagnosis of subarachnoid hemorrhage. Also, opening pressure and protein are often elevated with subarachnoid hemorrhage, but usually are not elevated with traumatic tap.

After the fluid is collected, the needle should be removed without the stylet in place; this eliminates the risk of compressing a nerve root and drawing the nerve root out as the needle is removed.

Patients may develop post-LP headache, manifested as severe headache that has an immediate onset after assuming the upright posture; lying down often relieves it. Allowing patients to lie down with legs up as fluids are consumed can relieve some of these headaches. This posture allows the dural hole to close, removing the source of spinal fluid leak. If the patient's assuming this posture for 72 hours does not cure the headache, an epidural patch with autologous blood taken from the patient's arm vein can be placed, usually by an anesthesiologist. Patients with coagulopathies may develop spinal epidural or subdural hematoma after LP; this can cause cauda equina compression. LP without aseptic technique may lead to infection of the site or osteomyelitis. Rarely, patients with raised intracranial pressure from a mass lesion may develop herniation after LP.

## SPINAL X-RAYS

Spinal x-rays evaluate patients inside or outside the hospital with neck and back pain, fractures and subluxations after trauma to the spine, destructive lesions associated with metastatic cancer to the spine (often in combination with bone scan), epidural abscess or osteomyelitis, overgrowth of Paget's disease, and spinal misalignment. Spinal x-rays are not useful for diagnosing soft-tissue injuries or disk herniations. Magnetic resonance imaging (MRI) provides more information about soft tissues and disk than x-rays and is especially useful in patients with cancer or epidural lesions. History of potential pregnancy must be obtained before x-rays are taken. Patients with reproductive potential should be appropriately shielded.

**PEARL: If patients have neck or head trauma, the neck should *not* be moved until full views of the cervical spine are obtained and completely evaluated to rule out instability. If the cervical spine has been injured and the neck is manipulated, cervical cord injury may occur or worsen.**

## SKULL X-RAYS

Computed tomography scanning has replaced skull x-rays for assessing skull fractures. Skull x-rays can help to assess potential facial fractures, traumatic and infectious lesions of the sinuses and orbits, or the bony disease of myeloma or Paget's disease.

## COMPUTED TOMOGRAPHY SCAN

**PEARL: In the emergency room, CT scan of the brain is the test of choice for virtually all neurologic disorders.** CT is useful in patients with various acute and chronic brain lesions (Table 2–2). CT

### Table 2–2. DISORDERS SEEN ON COMPUTED TOMOGRAPHY SCAN*

Ischemia and infarction

Acute and chronic intracerebral and subarachnoid hemorrhage

Arteriovenous malformation*

Abscess†

Tumor,† tumor-related edema, shift, and hydrocephalus

Atrophy of degenerative disorders

Subdural and epidural hematoma, contusions, intracranial air, fracture

Small and large ventricles

Carcinomatous meningitis*

---

*Note that several disorders listed here also appear in Table 2–3. The sensitivity and resolution provided by MRI exceed those of CT for these disorders.

†Detection improved with use of enhancing dyes (contrast).

scanning can also be performed after myelography to evaluate compressive lesions of the spinal cord or enlargement of the spinal cord. For the critically ill patient and for finding calcium or bone injury, CT is superior to MRI. However, artifact from bone may obscure scan results, especially when searching for subtle lesions in the posterior fossa. Issues of x-ray exposure apply to CT scanning. The patient must be able to lie flat and relatively still. Patients with reproductive potential should be appropriately shielded.

Dye, or "contrast," may be used to help highlight areas of blood-brain barrier disruption seen with vascular, infectious, and malignant lesions. Iodinated dye is used. It may be ionic or nonionic and crosses the blood-brain barrier. Ionic dyes are hypertonic; nonionic dyes are isotonic and hypoallergenic and induce less fluid overload or renal dysfunction. The incidence of fatal allergic reactions to either kind of dye is identical. The choice of dye used for a particular scan is made by the radiologist supervising the procedure. Aside from x-ray exposure, the typical neurology patient should have no specific complications associated with CT scan.

## MAGNETIC RESONANCE IMAGING

Magnetic resonance imaging has resolution superior to CT. Bone artifact is eliminated, thus rendering improved images of the posterior fossa and brainstem. **PEARL: MRI is the nonemergent test of choice for most central nervous system (CNS) lesions in neurology inpatients and outpatients (Table 2–3).** MRI with contrast is the noninvasive test of choice for diagnosing metastatic and primary tumors of the spinal cord, for evaluating spinal trauma after spinal x-rays are obtained, and if suspected, for diagnosing dural arteriovenous malformations and arteriovenous fistulas.

Anxiolytics may be needed before MRI in patients with claustrophobia. Patients who are critically ill and intubated may not be able to undergo MRI because a special ventilator with nonparamagnetic parts must be available. Patients with pacemakers, most aneurysm clips, and metal clips in visceral organs unimbedded in bone cannot undergo MRI, nor can critically ill patients who require continuous observation, because they cannot be easily observed by medical personnel during the procedure. These disadvantages make CT scanning the noninvasive test of choice for many acute brain injuries, including stroke and acute head trauma.

Shielding is unnecessary for MRI. Appropriate consent needs to be obtained from women of childbearing age or pregnant women, although there is

### Table 2–3. DISORDERS SEEN ON
### MAGNETIC RESONANCE IMAGING*

Acute and chronic imaging of small infarcts and posterior fossa infarcts

Hemorrhages present for days or weeks

Cavernous angiomas, arteriovenous malformations, and large aneurysms

Abscess

Tumor (advantageous for small posterior fossa tumors, isodense infiltrating gliomas, and meningeal carcinomatosis)

Atrophy of degenerative disorders

Subdural hematoma, diffuse axonal shearing injuries, contusions

Ventricular abnormalities, carcinomatous meningitis

Mesial temporal sclerosis

Cortical dysplasia and demyelinating lesions

Lesions of the craniocervical junction

Intervertebral disk disease

Intrinsic spinal cord lesions (demyelination, tumor, hemorrhages, infarction, syrinx, and trauma)

*Note that several disorders listed on Table 2–2 are also listed here. The sensitivity and resolution provided by MRI exceed those of CT for these disorders.

no evidence that MRI harms the fetus. The dye (gadolinium) used in MRI is not ionic. It highlights lesions that are associated with breakdown of the blood-brain barrier, helps distinguish tumor border from edema, determines activity in demyelinating lesions, and identifies isodense meningiomas. In spinal MRI, only the cervical, thoracic, or lumbosacral cord can be imaged in one sitting with great detail. A survey study of the entire spine can be performed, but it does not produce the detail of a focused spinal study. Survey studies are used when the entire space must be urgently imaged to rule out gross spinal cord compression.

# MYELOGRAPHY

Myelography is performed most often in outpatients who come to the hospital specifically for this test to evaluate degenerative disease of the spine when CT and MRI do not yield a clear diagnosis. The resolution of MRI is superior to myelography, but MRI often overestimates the true degree of spinal compression. A myelogram is superior to MRI or CT for establishing the true degree of spinal cord or root compression by disk or osteophyte and can detect cord arteriovenous malformations, epidural abscesses, and tumor. Myelography is more useful for identifying extramedullary lesions than for intramedullary spinal cord tumors. Preparation is similar to that for LP.

Performance is similar to LP except that the myelogram patient undergoes an LP in the prone position with fluoroscopic guidance for needle placement. The dye is a special iodinated, nonionic dye that is safe to instill into the subarachnoid space in direct contact with the spinal cord and nerve roots. A sample of CSF should be checked, as well as the opening and closing pressures in certain patients.

Complications are the same as for LP. **PEARL: Patients with large mass lesions producing spinal block may deteriorate neurologically after LP, as reduced pressure below the lesion following puncture leads to tissue shift and exacerbation of the clinical deficit.**

# ELECTROENCEPHALOGRAPHY

Electroencephalography (EEG) is commonly performed in all settings: emergency room, inpatient ward, and office. EEG measures brain electrical activity and helps to evaluate patients with seizures (both ictally and interictally); brain death; metabolic encephalopathy; and multifocal brain lesions such as those from dialysis, dementia, Creutzfeldt-Jakob disease, and herpes simplex encephalitis. It is also used to evaluate psychogenic coma.

Patients are told that wires and gel will be placed in their hair and that they may be required to be sleep deprived or have special electrodes placed before the procedure. Patients lie flat in a comfortable position and may be asked to hyperventilate or may be exposed to flashing lights to ascertain the electrophysiologic response. Nonspecific abnormalities include focal or diffuse slow waves (decreased frequency of brain waves), which may result from structural, metabolic, or physiologic disorders. Epileptiform abnormalities include sharp waves and spikes, which are strongly associated with epilepsy but are not, by themselves, diagnostic. A seizure is rarely recorded during EEG.

## ELECTROMYOGRAPHY

Electromyography (EMG) is a direct needle test of muscle, most often performed on outpatients. Fibrillations, positive sharp waves, loss of motor units, and polyphasic long-duration motor unit potentials (MUPs) suggest acute or subacute denervation. After nerve injury, 2 to 3 weeks must pass before these signs appear. Chronic denervation is characterized by large-amplitude MUPs, with increased duration and diminished MUP recruitment. These changes reflect collateral innervation, which occurs several months after nerve injury. Decreased amplitude and short duration of MUPs suggest muscle disease.

Nerve conduction velocity (NCV) studies can be performed on motor or sensory nerves. The sensory nerves that may be tested are the medial, ulnar, and radial nerves of the upper extremity and the sural, saphenous, superficial peroneal, and lateral femoral cutaneous nerves of the lower extremity. Motor NCVs of the facial nerve and upper and lower extremity nerves may be tested. NCV results are normal or only slightly diminished with disorders of the nerve axons, muscle, and neuromuscular junction. However, the amplitude of the potential is low. NCV is slowed significantly with myelin disorders.

The **F response** is a motor response obtained by distal stimulation of motor axons. This test measures the time an electric signal takes to travel antidromically (in reverse) along a motor nerve and return orthodromically to the muscle fibers. No synapse is involved. The response may be abnormal in patients with neuropathy.

The **H-reflex** is like a deep tendon reflex; the signal traverses a sensory nerve, synapse, and motor nerve. The soleus muscle is typically tested. The H-reflex is absent or prolonged in patients with S1 radiculopathy or neuropathy.

Nerve biopsy is seldom indicated in patients with polyneuropathy or mononeuritis multiplex. Patients suspected of having inflammatory disease (e.g., vasculitis, sarcoidosis), storage disease (e.g., amyloidosis, metachromatic leukodystrophy), or infectious disease (e.g., leprosy) may undergo nerve biopsy. Muscle biopsy is commonly performed in patients with muscle disease.

# 3
CHAPTER

# *Differential Diagnosis*

## CATEGORIES OF NEUROLOGIC ILLNESS

The history should help you to formulate a differential diagnosis. In every case, consider these categories of disease etiologies systematically:

Congenital
Developmental
Vascular (includes migraine)
Neoplastic (primary or metastatic)
Traumatic
Systemic-toxic (organ failure, metabolic derangements, treatment-induced)
Hereditary
Degenerative
Infectious
Inflammatory
Autoimmune
Demyelinating
Epileptic
Iatrogenic
Psychiatric/functional

# TIME COURSE OF
# NEUROLOGIC ILLNESS

**PEARL: The tempo of the illness over time will often delimit possible etiologies.** When was the earliest neurologic symptom and how did the disorder evolve? For example, congenital disorders are static with time. Degenerative and neoplastic diseases are usually insidious in onset and relentlessly progressive. However, a metastatic lesion may present a strokelike onset when there is bleeding into a high-grade glioma with herniation or hydrocephalus.

A **paroxysmal** time course is consistent with a seizure disorder, migraine headaches, or the "on-off" phenomenon of Parkinson's disease. Abrupt onset of deficits with a monophasic course is consistent with traumatic, vascular, structural, and infectious etiologies. **Polyphasic** courses suggest inflammatory and metabolic causes. An acute or subacute but progressive course with fever suggests infection. There are many exceptions to these temporal patterns, however, such as paroxysmal symptoms in multiple sclerosis, the abrupt onset of a deficit with a tumor, or a stuttering course in ischemic strokes.

The family history may suggest a genetic diathesis or subtle stigmata of neurologic disease in family members. Ask about consanguinity. If the patient is left-handed, lack of family history suggests a possible pathologic left-handedness (early left hemisphere insult).

# THE IMPORTANCE OF FINDING
# TREATABLE DISORDERS

**PEARL: The final differential diagnosis should summarize the most likely site or sites of localization and**

**list two or three leading possibilities.** Your assessment and plan should follow logically from the facts documented in the history and exam. An independent reviewer should arrive at a similar endpoint.

The diagnostic work-up should "clinch" the leading diagnosis and must emphasize the most treatable etiologies. For example, even when the history and exam are strongly consistent with motor neuron disease as the cause of a degenerative spastic paraparesis, make every effort to consider and exclude cervical spondylosis, demyelinating disease, or $B_{12}$ deficiency.

**PEARL: When an untreatable disorder is the leading diagnosis, investigate and treat any complicating non-neurologic conditions.** For example, a urinary tract infection or adverse medication effect may account for sudden deterioration in an otherwise stable patient with classic signs of Alzheimer's disease.

## DIAGNOSTIC EVALUATION AND FOLLOW-UP

If the neurologic exam is normal, state so. **PEARL: The assessment of "no neurologic disease" is often more valuable and comforting than the detection of subtle focality.** To acquire the confidence that an exam is normal and to get a feel for the range of normal, you should examine at least as many patients with normal findings as those with known disease. If you have doubts about a diagnosis, decide an interval for follow-up exams. Time is the neurologist's best diagnostic assistant.

When arranging diagnostic evaluations, avoid formulaic work-ups. The cost-benefit ratio in testing for neurologic disorders is coming under greater scrutiny. Consider the sensitivity, specificity, yield, cost, and risks of neurodiagnostic testing. Be prepared to justify how the result of each test will influence your differential diagnosis or treatment decisions.

**PEARL: When consulting other specialists, including neuroradiologists, or scheduling lab tests, ask *specific* questions.** It reflects on your clinical acumen and is a basic professional courtesy. The quality of the interpretation you will get is related directly to the information provided to your consultant. For example, do not order "EMG/NCV"—instead, ask, "Is there a sensorimotor polyneuropathy versus root lesion at L4?" Do not request "Cervical spine MRI"—ask, "History and exams suggest left C6 root lesion likely due to spondylosis versus tumor." Your consultants will respect your professionalism and give you interpretations of greater quality.

**PEARL: Define *target* symptoms that will monitor the outcome of your therapeutic maneuvers and address these at each follow-up visit.** Include brief documentation of warnings or advice given to the patient. Document that the "risks, benefits, and alternatives" have been explained to the patient and caregivers before initiating potentially hazardous diagnostic or therapeutic plans. Risk-prone items for neurologists are antiepileptics, benzodiazepines, corticosteroids, and anticoagulants.

# 2
PART

*Outpatient*
*Neurologic*
*Problems*

# 4

# *Headache and Face Pain*

**Primary headaches** are benign disorders that include migraine (without or with aura), tension-type headaches (episodic or chronic), cluster headaches, post-traumatic headaches, and drug-rebound headaches. **Secondary headaches** result from underlying organic disease. The brain is not sensitive to pain, but other tissues in the head and neck are densely innervated. Pain-sensitive structures include the scalp and its blood vessels, dura mater, the arteries of the meninges, larger cerebral arteries, the great venous and cranial sinuses, fibers of cranial nerves V, IX, and X and the upper cervical nerves, head and neck muscles, and other soft tissues in the head. Most benign headache disorders involve disturbances in the trigeminal and cranial nerve innervation of the meninges and vascular structures.

## APPROACH TO THE PATIENT WITH HEADACHE

Neurologic exam of the patient with headache is usually unremarkable, so diagnosis relies even

more heavily on a detailed history. Information to
elicit includes the following:

- *General health status:* Constitutional complaints (malaise, anorexia, weight loss) suggest organic disease. **PEARL: In older persons,
  headaches and constitutional symptoms with or
  without jaw claudication or visual disturbance
  suggest temporal arteritis until proved otherwise.**
- *Family history:* Genetic trends are prominent
  in migraines, particularly in hemiplegic migraine.
- *Age when headache first occurred:* Migraine
  headaches usually begin in childhood or ado-
  lescence. Onset of headaches in later life de-
  mands a rigorous search to exclude an organic cause.
- *Characteristics and location of headaches:*
  **PEARL: Headaches that are always on the same
  side are atypical for migraines and suggest a vascular malformation or structural lesion.**
- *Frequency:* **PEARL: Disabling headaches occurring more than twice a month are better managed by using prophylactic, rather than abortive,
  medicines.**
- *Duration of headaches:* Migraine and tension-
  type headaches continue for hours to days;
  cluster headaches last from minutes up to an
  hour.
- *Whether headaches are progressively worsening:* A qualitative or quantitative change in
  an established headache pattern mandates
  prompt investigation by neuroimaging.
- *Factors that trigger headaches:* Sleep deprivation and tyramine-rich foods trigger migraines. Alcohol is a common trigger of migraine and cluster headaches; stress provokes
  migraine and tension-type headaches.
- *Symptoms that precede or accompany headaches:* Classic migraines (migraine with aura)

are typically preceded by visual auras; nausea and vomiting rarely accompany tension-type headaches.

- *Aggravating factors:* During migraine episodes, patients are unusually sensitive to light **(photophobia)** or sound **(phonophobia).** They avoid physical exertion during an attack.
- *Severity of headaches:* In choosing among medicines with differing toxicities, the impact of headaches on social or vocational functioning must be considered.
- *Psychosocial history:* The patient's lifestyle, current stressors, and expectations of treatment outcomes must be explored.

Certain items in the clinical picture heighten suspicion of an organic cause:

- *Sudden onset of a new severe headache:* Subarachnoid hemorrhage due to a ruptured aneurysm is often described as "something snapped in my head" or "worst headache of my life."
- *Progressively worsening headache:* Intracranial mass lesions commonly have a pattern of progressive worsening.
- *Precipitation by exertion, coughing, straining, sexual intercourse, and positional change:* Dural tears, ruptured vascular malformations, and increased intracranial pressure may worsen with these maneuvers. Headaches caused by a colloid cyst in the third ventricle typically worsen when bending over and subside when sitting up. Cough- and coital-induced headaches are often benign disorders.
- *Awakening from sleep:* Headaches that disturb sleep or are most severe on arising in the morning suggest increased intracranial pressure or sleep apnea syndromes. Migraines may present similarly and are the most common cause of morning headache.

- *Impaired consciousness:* Drowsiness, confusion, or memory loss is not consistent with benign headache disorders.
- *Systemic complaints:* Chronic malaise, myalgia, or arthralgia suggests a systemic disorder as the cause of headache. Fever merits exclusion of a meningoencephalitis or parameningeal focus (e.g., sinusitis).
- *Progressive visual, motor, or balance disturbance:* Focal neurologic findings increase the likelihood of a tumor or vascular lesion.
- *Onset of headache after age 50:* Although benign headache syndromes may begin in middle age, temporal arteritis and intracranial lesions should be excluded.

The physical and neurologic exams seek signs of organic causes:

- *Vital signs:* fever, hypertension, tachycardia
- Impaired alertness
- *Meningeal irritation:* resistance to passive neck flexion; Kernig's or Brudzinski's sign
- Papilledema
- Pupil asymmetry or impaired reactivity
- Visual field loss, focal motor or sensory loss, anosmia
- Abnormal gait
- Indurated, tender temporal arteries
- Abnormal temporomandibular joint (TMJ) motion

## PRIMARY HEADACHE SYNDROMES

### Tension-Type Headache

**Tension-type headache** is the most common primary headache, accounting for 60% of headaches. These headaches are described as a diffuse, bilateral, bandlike, constant, constricting ache or pressure, often worsening at day's end. Tension-type and typical migraine headaches may co-exist. Patients are often depressed or anxious. There is usually no nausea, vomiting, photophobia, or phonophobia. Tension-type headaches usually occur fewer than 15 days per month. A chronic daily pattern may develop gradually. Although muscle tension occurs in these headaches, central mechanisms are more causal. Tension-type and migraine headaches comprise a continuum of neurovascular headaches, ranging between migraine with aura to daily tension-type headaches.

Treatment of tension-type headaches involves reassurance, counseling, regular exercise, biofeedback and stress management techniques, and the judicious use of tricyclic antidepressants. Infrequent tension-type headaches usually respond to acetaminophen or nonsteroidal anti-inflammatory agents. Chronic tension-type headaches may benefit from tramodol (25 to 50 mg every 4 to 6 hours). When anxiety is prominent, benzodiazepines (diazepam 2 mg p.o. bid or tid) may be useful.

## Migraine

Migraine headaches are reported in 18% of women and 6% of men. Women aged 30 to 49 years have the highest prevalence and frequency of migraines. Migraines cause moderate to severe disability in 50% of those who have them. More than half of patients with migraines go undiagnosed and self-prescribe over-the-counter medicines. **PEARL: Migraine is a "sick headache" producing recurrent, throbbing, unilateral or bilateral headaches.** Migraine attacks have five phases:

1. *Prodrome:* Patients may feel depressed, anxious, or elated. They may experience anorexia or food cravings.
2. *Aura:* Some patients experience an aura, usually visual, consisting of fortification spectra (e.g., zigzag lines) migrating across the visual field, a scintillating scotoma, or **photopsia** (flashing lights). **Sensory auras** (paresthesias or numbness) are the next most common; aphasia or unilateral motor weakness auras are rare. The aura reflects spreading cerebral depression and decreased cerebral perfusion. Auras generally develop gradually, over about 4 minutes, and rarely persist beyond an hour. Auras usually occur before the headache, but they can also occur during or even after it, or without any associated headache. Symptoms may very rarely be permanent, as a result of cerebral infarction. Unlike partial epilepsy, in which the march of symptoms lasts only seconds, in migraine it takes minutes. In **migraine without aura (common migraine),** headache pain is typically unilateral and pulsating in quality.
3. *Headache:* Patients experience severe pain with photophobia, phonophobia, **osmophobia** (sensitivity to a smell), anorexia, nausea, and vomiting. Patients take to bed and lie still, avoiding physical exertion. During the headache phase, cerebral hyperperfusion occurs, associated with sterile inflammation in meningeal vessels and large arteries. Vasoactive mediators are released and stimulate the trigeminovascular system, causing pain. Headaches can last up to 72 hours.
4. *Headache termination:* Migraines are relieved by abortive agents, rest in a dark room, or sleep.
5. *Postdrome:* Patients may feel malaise, depression, or exhaustion.

### *Triggers*

Migraine triggers should be sought, because modifying them may lessen headache frequency and severity. Triggers of migraine include:

- *Hormones:* sudden decreases in serum estradiol. Many women have more migraines with onset of menses and relief during pregnancy. **PEARL: Migraines generally improve after menopause, but they can sometimes worsen.**
- *Chronobiologic factors:* sleep deprivation, insomnia, jet lag.
- *Carbon monoxide.*
- *Sensory stimuli:* strong odors, deodorants, perfume.
- *Foods and beverages:* aged cheeses, red wines, chocolate, and preserved foods with a high tyramine content; monosodium glutamate, and aspartame.
- *Drugs:* nitrates and related vasodilators (e.g., sildenafil [Viagra]), ergot rebound.
- *Emotional stress.*

### *Diagnosis and Treatment*

Migraine is diagnosed clinically. If there has been a dramatic change in the character or severity of headaches, if the headaches have atypical features, or if focal neurologic signs are detected, imaging and lumbar puncture are used to exclude structural lesions and infections. **PEARL: Clinically, migraine is differentiated from tension-type headache by the longer headache duration, greater severity, pulsatile or throbbing pain quality, gastrointestinal (GI) distress, and predictable aggravation with physical activity.** The leading hypothesis for the origin of migraine is a neurovascular disturbance triggered by multiple stimuli having an impact on serotonin (5-hydroxytryptamine [5-HT]) transmission in the central nervous system

(CNS). Serotonin receptors modulate neurotransmitter release by cranial nerves, particularly the trigeminal nerve, and mediate neurogenic inflammation and pain.

*Treatment* involves elimination or modification of identifiable triggers. Oral contraceptives and estrogen replacement therapy may either exacerbate or ameliorate migraines. Strokes are increased in women with migraines who take oral contraceptives and smoke. *Abortive* treatments are considered for patients with infrequent headaches (generally fewer than three a month). Abortive medicines include **sumatriptan,** a 5-HT1$_D$ receptor agonist. Sumatriptan rapidly abolishes pain and accompanying symptoms of migraine (GI distress, photophobia, phonophobia) and is useful even after the headache is established. Sumatriptan can be given by subcutaneous routes (6 mg s.c.) and can be repeated once within 24 hours. Oral sumatriptan is available in 25- and 50-mg tablets; doses above 100 mg at the onset of headache are not more effective. Sumatriptan is also available as a nasal spray in 5 and 20 mg. Adverse effects of sumatripan include injection site reactions, paresthesias in the limbs, and chest pressure. It is contraindicated in patients with hemiplegic migraine, ischemic heart disease, uncontrolled hypertension, or those who have recently received ergotamines. The first dose of sumatriptan should be given under medical supervision. Many congeners of the triptan molecule are now appearing for oral use, with varying degrees of efficacy and a similar profile of adverse effects.

Ergotamine-caffeine (oral, sublingual, inhaled, or suppository) is another abortive medicine. One to two tablets are taken orally, with a maximum of 5 tablets per attack and 10 tablets per week. Mixed preparations of ergots with caffeine are available, as are suppositories and inhalational preparations. Contraindications to ergots include pregnancy; hypertension; and renal, hepatic, peripheral, coronary, or cerebrovascular disease. Dihydroergotamine (DHE-45) is an effective abortive agent (0.5 mg i.v., i.m., or s.c. every 4 hours) with contraindications similar to those for ergotamine. DHE-45 is less prone to induce vasoconstriction and is about as effective as sumatriptan in reducing neurogenic inflammation. DHE frequently produces nausea, and patients should receive metaclopramide 10 mg i.v. before each DHE dose. DHE is available as a nasal spray.

Other abortive agents include combination medicines such as Extra-Strength Excedrin, butalbital-aspirin-caffeine or butalbital-acetaminophen-caffeine, antiemetics (prochlorperazine), anxiolytics, nonsteroidal anti-inflammatory drugs (NSAIDs), corticosteroids, isometheptene (Midrin), and major tranquilizers (chlorpromazine).

In general, opioids should be avoided. Butorphanol is a mixed opioid agonist-antagonist with a low liability for addiction or dependence. It is available as a nasal spray, given as one sniff at onset of headache; this may be repeated in 1 hour. Common side effects include nasal irritation, drowsiness, dizziness, and confusion. **PEARL: Diluting butorphanol with normal saline will lessen its adverse effects while retaining efficacy.**

**Status migrainosus** (severe, unrelenting attacks associated with nausea and vomiting, lasting more than 72 hours) may require hospitalization for vigorous fluid repletion and can be treated with methylprednisolone 60 to 80 mg/day i.v., or DHE 0.5 mg and metaclopramide 10 mg i.v. every 4 to 6 hours.

### *Prophylaxis*

**PEARL: *Prophylaxis* should be considered for patients having two to three incapacitating attacks**

**per month (or even one severe, prolonged episode monthly), for patients who are unable to tolerate abortive medicines, and for patients psychologically disabled by headaches.** *Beta-blockers* are effective prophylactic agents. Propranolol is most effective, probably because of its high CNS penetrance. Doses up to 480 mg daily can be used, and sustained-release forms are available. Other useful beta-blockers include nadolol, atenolol, metoprolol, and timolol. Patients should be screened for relative contraindications, including chronic obstructive pulmonary disease, asthma, congestive heart failure, uncontrolled diabetes, and peripheral vascular disease.

*Valproic acid* is approved for migraine prophylaxis. Divided doses totaling 500 to 3000 mg/day are effective. Blood levels document compliance or toxicity but are not clearly correlated with efficacy. Common adverse effects include weight gain, hair loss, nausea, or drowsiness.

*Calcium channel blockers* are sometimes effective. Verapamil, diltiazam, and nifedipine have been tried. Verapamil is given in doses of 80 to 240 mg daily; hypotension and constipation are limiting side effects.

*Tricyclic antidepressants* are effective. They include amitryptiline, nortryptiline, doxepin, and imipramine. Side effects of the tricyclics may be used to therapeutic advantage; for example, if insomnia is prominent, the more sedating amitryptiline or doxepin might be chosen. Effective doses range from 10 to 150 mg daily. *Selective serotonin reuptake inhibitors,* such as fluoxetine, can rarely be helpful but occasionally worsen headaches.

*Ciproheptadine* (8 to 32 mg p.o. qd in divided doses) is an antihistamine that produces drowsiness. *Methysergide* (2 mg tid or qid) is an underused prophylactic agent, but because it can occasionally produce severe fibrotic disease after 6 months of continuous use, it should be stopped every 5 months for 1 month to avoid retroperitoneal, cardiac, and pulmonary fibrosis.

*Aspirin* (325 mg p.o. qd) and related nonsteroidal anti-inflammatory agents are useful. When these agents are prescribed chronically or in high doses, serious GI hemorrhage may occur, however.

**PEARL: When prescribing prophylactic medicines for migraine, the initial agent should be chosen by considering concurrent conditions.** For example, a tricyclic antidepressant is useful for a patient with depression, but an NSAID might be preferable with concurrent arthritis. Monotherapy should be sought whenever possible. The therapeutic expectation that headaches will be reduced, but not eliminated entirely, should be explained, as well as common adverse effects. Agents should be tried sequentially and pushed to effectiveness or clear toxicity. **PEARL: Patients on prophylaxis should always receive abortive medicines for "breakthrough" headaches.**

*Nonpharmacologic approaches* to migraine are worthwhile: Identifying and eliminating dietary and lifestyle triggers and biofeedback are effective. Stress management techniques, regular exercise, and good sleeping habits should be emphasized.

## Drug-Rebound Headache

Excessive analgesic use by patients prone to migraine or tension-type headaches may cause the under-recognized syndrome of rebound, chronic daily headache, or drug-induced headache. Clinical features include a constant, diffuse, bilateral headache associated with GI complaints and photosensitivity, usually worsened by mild physical or mental exertion. Patients may awaken in the early morning with headache and complain of constant restlessness, impaired memory or concentration, nausea, asthenia, and depression. Work and social habits become dysfunctional. To fend off rebound headaches, patients consume excessive amounts of medicines containing barbiturates, opioids, and caffeine. In this syndrome, prophylactic therapy fails. Treatment usually requires inpatient detoxification. Rebound headaches are managed by stopping all migraine medicines and providing vigorous hydration and a scheduled regimen of DHE (0.5 to 1 mg i.v. every 8 hours), along with metoclopramide 10 mg i.v. Concomitant anxiety is quelled by benzodiazepines as necessary. Most patients detoxify within several days and then become available for lifestyle counseling and prophylactic regimens.

## Cluster Headaches

Cluster headaches usually occur in middle-aged men and manifest as severe, unilateral pain, lasting minutes to hours, typically at night. Pain localizes to the eye, temple, forehead, and cheek. "Cluster" refers to the daily occurrence of symptoms over a period of weeks to months, followed by a temporary remission lasting months or years. On exam, there may be Horner's syndrome, facial sweating, eyelid edema, conjunctival injection, and rhinorrhea. Unlike patients with migraines, who prefer to remain quiet, patients with cluster headaches pace the floor in agony or pound their heads with their fists. The diagnosis is clinical. Acute closed-angle glaucoma is the most important differential diagnosis to consider; measuring intraocular pressure at the time of the headache excludes this ophthalmologic emergency. Carotid dissection also should be considered. Headache onset is often too rapid and transient for effective abortive therapy. However, relief is gained by inhaling oxygen via nasal cannula (greater than 7 L/min for 5 to 10 minutes), from parenteral or nasal dihydroergotamine or sumatriptan, or from short-acting opioids. (See the preceding discussion of migraine for contraindications and other information.)

Prophylactic treatment during the cluster headache period includes methysergide (4 to 8 mg p.o. qd in divided doses). As mentioned in regard to migraine prophylaxis, it should be stopped every 5 months for 1 month. Other prophylactic agents include ergotamine tartrate (one tablet bid), lithium (300 to 1200 mg/day p.o. in divided doses), verapamil (80 to 240 mg/day in divided doses), corticosteroids (e.g., prednisone 40 mg/day with gradual taper), and intranasal lidocaine.

## Chronic Paroxysmal Hemicrania

Chronic paroxysmal hemicrania occurs mostly in women and consists of severe unilateral head pains, typically lasting 15 to 30 minutes. The attacks occur 15 to 30 times daily. Pain is localized to the temple, forehead, ear, eye, or occipital regions and may be accompanied by lacrimation, rhinorrhea, ptosis, and conjunctival injection. Neck movements may provoke these headaches, unlike cluster headaches. These headaches are exquisitely responsive to indomethacin.

## Benign Intracranial Hypertension

Benign intracranial hypertension produces diffuse, fairly constant headaches occasionally associated with transient visual obscurations in one or both eyes. Patients are typically obese, hirsute-appearing young women, but the disorder is also associated with corticosteroids, excessive vitamin A therapy, tetracycline, nitrofurantoin, and oral contraceptive use. Endocrine studies are normal. The exam often reveals papilledema, loss of venous pulsations, an enlarged blind spot, and occasionally unilateral or bilateral sixth nerve palsy from intracranial hypertension (false localizing sign). Computed tomography (CT) and magnetic resonance imaging (MRI) scans are normal, or reveal slitlike ventricles. Neuroimaging studies will exclude dural venous thrombosis, which may mimic benign intracranial hypertension. In atypical cases, cerebral angiography may be required. Lumbar puncture reveals an elevated opening pressure, typically above 250 mm of cerebrospinal fluid (CSF), with a normal CSF profile or low protein. After removing CSF, the closing pressure declines to the normal range. Often, the first lumbar puncture results in a prolonged remission of headache. Repeated punctures, performed daily or less often and reducing opening pressures to normal, may successfully control the syndrome. Patients must be followed up regularly by quantitative perimetry. Persistent headache or compromised visual fields are indications for more aggressive therapy, which may include carbonic anhydrase inhibitors (acetazolamide), corticosteroids, optic nerve sheath fenestration, or lumboperitoneal shunt.

## SECONDARY HEADACHES

### Mass Lesions (Tumors, Subdural Hematoma)

Daily, progressive headache is the cardinal sign of *mass lesions*. There may be early morning awakening by the headache, with nausea and vomiting. Pain is usually described as dull and nonpulsatile. It can be intermittent or steady and worsens with postural changes and exertion. With *intra-axial lesions*, focal signs are typically more prominent than reduced level of consciousness. With *extra-axial lesions*, such as subdural hematoma, an impaired level of alertness typically exceeds the severity of any focal signs, and may fluctuate. Imaging tests verify the diagnosis; MRI is the best initial choice. In an emergency setting (e.g., herniation), a noncontrast CT to direct initial therapies is usually more accessible and can be completed more rapidly. For primary therapy, refer to Chapter 21.

## Temporal Arteritis

Symptoms and signs of *temporal arteritis* include diffuse or temporal headaches associated with constitutional complaints of fever, anorexia, malaise, weight loss, and anemia. Dreaded complications include blindness and, less commonly, cranial neuropathy and stroke. Once present, vision loss is usually permanent. Occasionally patients describe jaw claudication due to ischemia in the facial arteries. Complaints of transient visual loss **(amaurosis fugax)** are ominous, preceding irreversible visual loss. Patients at risk of temporal arteritis are typically elderly, more often women. There is an overlap between temporal arteritis and the more benign *polymyalgia rheumatica*. The exam discloses tender, indurated temporal arteries and pale optic disks due to anterior ischemic optic neuropathy. When polymyalgia co-exists, there is intensely severe aching in the shoulder and hip girdle. Patients have a markedly elevated erythrocyte sedimentation rate (ESR)—usually more than 50 mm/h. Temporal arteritis rarely occurs in younger persons, but "a sed rate over 50 in a patient over 50" is a useful diagnostic pearl.

**PEARL: Temporal arteritis is a treatable neurologic emergency.** High-dose corticosteroids (e.g., prednisone 100 mg p.o. qd) should be started on clinical grounds in conjunction with an elevated ESR and should *not* be deferred pending temporal artery biopsy. Unilateral temporal artery biopsy is positive in only half of cases. Steroid therapy is tapered over months up to a year while the ESR and constitutional symptoms are monitored. Daily therapy is required. Methotrexate offers "steroid-sparing" anti-inflammatory benefits and is particularly useful for elderly patients susceptible to steroid complications.

## Post-Traumatic Headache

**Post-traumatic headache** (postconcussion syndrome) occurs following minor head trauma, or even after abrupt cervical hyperextension-flexion injury ("whiplash") without direct trauma to the head. Diffuse, constant headaches start in the first days after injury. They may throb or be steady and are associated with complaints of impaired attention, concentration, and memory. The patient is irritable, dizzy, vertiginous, nauseated, and emotionally labile. Patients sometimes report "blackouts," but syncope or seizures are not observed. Headaches typically remit over weeks to months. **PEARL: The results of neurologic exam and imaging studies are normal in post-traumatic headaches.** If seizures are absent, electroencephalography is not useful. Most patients improve when reassured they have a genuine biologic syndrome that will eventually resolve. Some patients go on to develop recurrent migraine or tension-type headaches. Tricyclics (in doses similar to those for migraine prophylaxis) help to improve sleep and to reduce headache severity and any associated anxiety or depression.

## Temporomandibular Joint Dysfunction

*Temporomandibular joint dysfunction* is associated with preauricular pains radiating to the ear or jaw, worsened by chewing. It is a steady, unilateral ache, more often seen in edentulous patients. The joint may be tender, and crepitus on movement may be detected. There may be an associated spasm of masseter or pterygoid muscles. **PEARL: TMJ is overdiagnosed as a cause of headache and facial pain. Diagnosis is made clinically: Pain is reproduced by specific movements of the jaw or by palpation of its muscles and ligaments.** Selective anesthetic blocks help to corroborate the diagnosis. Imaging procedures delineate joint pathology (degenerative change, dislocation). An experienced dentist or otolaryngologist best manages treatment. Treatment modalities include a soft diet, application of heat or ice, NSAIDs, an occlusal orthotic, and physical therapy.

## ACUTE HEADACHE SYNDROMES

### Subarachnoid Hemorrhage

A cardinal symptom of *subarachnoid hemorrhage* is sudden onset of severe headache, with or without loss of consciousness, often associated with neck stiffness in flexion. For most patients, a reduced level of consciousness is more prominent than focal signs such as cranial nerve palsy and hemiparesis. If performed within 24 hours after onset of bleeding, noncontrast CT scan can detect as little as 5 mL of blood in the subarachnoid space in nearly all patients and often points to the source of hemorrhage from an aneurysm.

Lumbar puncture typically reveals an elevated opening pressure and numerous red blood cells. To distinguish true subarachnoid hemorrhage from traumatic lumbar puncture, the *last* tube of CSF collected should be immediately centrifuged, and its supernatant checked for xanthochromia. Xanthochromia begins about 2 hours after subarachnoid hemorrhage and is absent in a traumatic lumbar puncture when the supernatant is examined immediately. MRI may demonstrate flow voids in aneurysms or arteriovenous malformations. Four-vessel angiography remains the gold standard for diagnosis and reveals an aneurysm in most cases of spontaneous nontraumatic subarachnoid hemorrhage; one-tenth as often, a vascular malformation is discovered. Treatment is discussed in Chapter 19.

## Meningitis

Compared with subarachnoid hemorrhage, the headache of *meningitis* is gradual in onset and is associated with neck stiffness in flexion, photophobia, malaise, nausea, vomiting, and fever. **PEARL: When acute meningitis is suspected, never delay lumbar puncture while awaiting the outcome of neuroimaging studies.** If raised intracranial pressure or papilledema is present, treat these as the lumbar puncture is initiated. Lumbar puncture and CSF analysis will suggest whether the etiology is likely to be viral, bacterial, fungal, inflammatory, or neoplastic. In bacterial meningitis or herpes meningoencephalitis, neurologic recovery is best correlated with rapid treatment. The primary source of infection (e.g., sinusitis, pneumonia) is treated.

## Sinusitis

Patients with *sinusitis* have headaches associated with nasal discharge and, occasionally, fever and tenderness of the sinuses. Many benign headache syndromes are wrongly ascribed to sinusitis. The clinical picture is often diagnostic. Plain films (sinus series), CT, or MRI demonstrate fluid collections in the sinuses. Antibiotics, with or without surgical drainage, are indicated.

## Glaucoma

*Acute closed-angle glaucoma* produces headache and retro-orbital pain associated with redness and congestion in the affected eye. Nausea and vomiting may be present. The eye may feel tense to palpation, with optic atrophy and crescentic visual field deficits. Diagnosis is suspected clinically and verified by measuring intraocular pressures. **PEARL: Acute angle-closure glaucoma is an ophthalmologic emergency.**

## Post–Lumbar Puncture Headache

See Chapter 2.

## FACIAL PAIN

## Trigeminal Neuralgia

*Trigeminal neuralgia* (*tic douloureux*), more common in women and in older patients, is suggested by severe, paroxysmal, unilateral facial pains. Patients report brief, lancinating, shocklike, jabbing or sharp pains lasting seconds to minutes. The neurologic exam results are normal. This syndrome can be idiopathic or caused by tortuous brainstem vessels irritating the trigeminal roots in the posterior fossa.

The cheek, lips, gums, and chin (V2 and V3 territories) are more often affected than the forehead or eye (V1 territory). Trigger points may develop. Light touch, cold breezes, chewing, shaving, speaking, or brushing teeth often precipitates pain. Fewer than 10% of patients have bilateral tics. Frequency of attacks varies from sporadic to many per day, and for several minutes after a paroxysm, the patient is often refractory to further episodes. Attacks typically increase in frequency and severity over a period of years, but occasional remissions may be encountered. Symptoms are often attributed to dental pathology, delaying the diagnosis. Diagnosis may be made clinically. Multiple sclerosis should be suspected in young patients, particularly with bilateral tic. MRI is recommended in all cases to rule out demyelination in younger patients, or if a mass lesion (e.g., neuroma, meningioma) is suspected in older patients.

Most patients with trigeminal neuralgia benefit from medical therapy. First-line therapy is carbamazepine 200 to 1600 mg p.o. per day in divided doses, which often provides dramatic relief. Alternative choices include phenytoin 300 to 600 mg daily p.o. in divided doses; clonazepam 4 to 6 mg per day in divided doses; baclofen 40 to 80 mg per day p.o. in divided doses; or pimozide 1 to 2 mg per day p.o. in divided doses. Recently, gabapentin (up to 3600 mg/day in divided doses) has been found useful. In refractory cases, combinations of these medicines should be tried.

As the disorder progresses, medical therapy may falter and surgical options must often be considered. Percutaneous alcohol or glycerin ganglionolysis, rhizotomy, or radiofrequency coagulation of the trigeminal ganglion or its roots are all effective but may be complicated by facial numbness, corneal anesthesia, or "painful numbness" **(anesthesia dolorosa)**. Repositioning of tortuous brainstem vessels (anterior inferior cerebellar artery) by the Janetta procedure requires a suboccipital craniotomy. **PEARL: Gamma knife radiation of the trigeminal ganglion is the newest modality reported to benefit medically refractory patients with trigeminal neuralgia.**

## Glossopharyngeal Neuralgia

*Glossopharyngeal neuralgia* is much less common than trigeminal neuralgia. Unilateral paroxysms of lancinating pain occur in the distribution of the glossopharyngeal and vagus nerves, affecting the jaw, ear, oropharynx, or tongue; pain radiates from the oropharynx to the ear. There may be deep, continuing pain between attacks. Coughing, swallowing, drinking, chewing, talking, and yawning may precipitate episodes. The neurologic exam results are normal. A rare patient experiences bradycardia, syncope, or asystole during an episode. Tumors involving the lower cranial nerves around the jugular foramen should be excluded by neuroimaging. Medical treatments are similar to those for trigeminal neuralgia. Intracranial sectioning of cranial nerve IX and the upper rootlets of cranial nerve X at the jugular foramen should be considered in refractory cases.

## Occipital Neuralgia

**Occipital neuralgia** presents as continuous or paroxysmal pain arising from the occipitocervical junction, radiating superiorly to the vertex. There may be reduced sensation and paresthesias in the territory of the greater and lesser occipital nerves, along with local tenderness. In the elderly patient, cervical spondylosis with nerve entrapment is a common cause. Cervical spine radiographs are often sufficiently diagnostic. These patients are managed with a cervical collar and simple analgesics. Younger patients without definite pathology may benefit from a brief course of steroids, nonsteroidal analgesics, or anticonvulsants.

## Atypical Trigeminal Neuralgia

Patients with **atypical trigeminal neuralgia** have persistent facial pain over a prolonged period, rather than in paroxysms. Patients may have severe paroxysms of pain superimposed on sensory symptoms and abnormal findings on sensory exam. Because the likelihood of a structural abnormality is increased in this setting, definitive investigation is required. MRI and lumbar puncture exclude multiple sclerosis, tumors, and meningitides. Emotional and psychological factors must be explored. If no secondary cause is found, treatment is identical to that for typical neuralgia. Occasionally, tricyclic antidepressants and anticonvulsants (e.g., gabapentin) prove beneficial. If a secondary cause is found, patients are still treated symptomatically but the primary cause must be addressed.

## Trigeminal Neuropathy

Patients with **trigeminal neuropathy** experience constant numbness in the distribution of the trigeminal nerve. Paroxysmal pain may be superimposed. Exam findings are abnormal, with sensory impairment or an abnormal corneal reflex. Differential diagnoses include tumor (nasopharyngeal carcinoma, neurinoma, metastasis, acoustic schwannoma), multiple sclerosis, connective tissue disease (scleroderma, mixed connective tissue disease), and sarcoidosis. Sensory neuropathy of the chin (mental neuropathy) results from CNS lymphoma or metastasis. About 20% of cases are idiopathic. MRI, lumbar puncture, and serologic tests for vasculitis or infection are indicated. Idiopathic cases of trigeminal neuropathy may remit spontaneously. For patients with trigeminal neuropathy due to other causes, treat the primary problem. Carbamazepine and gabapentin may help.

## Atypical Facial Pain

Patients with *atypical facial pain* are typically much younger than those with trigeminal neuralgia or trigeminal neuropathy. The disorder is more common in women. The symptoms include constant unilateral or bilateral facial pain. The pain is deep, continuous, and sometimes burning in quality. No triggers or precipitants are described. Exam findings are normal. Many patients have underlying affective or thought disorders, particularly depression. In addition to the evaluation outlined above for atypical trigeminal neuralgia and trigeminal neuropathy, these patients should be evaluated by a specialist in TMJ disorders. The primary cause should be treated. Some patients respond to antidepressants.

## INCREASED INTRACRANIAL PRESSURE

## Anatomy and Pathophysiology

The cranium houses the meninges, brain, blood, and CSF. **PEARL: Any *increase* in the amount of blood, CSF, or brain volume (e.g., edema) must be**

**compensated for by a *decrease* in other intracranial constituents and will raise intracranial pressure.** The increased pressure may result from:

- Focal or diffuse disorders that lead to increased intracranial volume (e.g., frontal tumor, subdural hematoma, acute brain swelling from anoxia)
- Disorders of CSF flow or absorption (e.g., obstructive hydrocephalus, choroid plexus papillomas)
- Venous obstruction (e.g., superior sagittal sinus thrombosis, jugular or superior vena cava occlusion) or high venous back pressure (e.g., heart failure)

## Clinical Features

Clinical features characteristic of increased intracranial pressure include:

- Headache
- Nausea and vomiting
- Lethargy
- Double vision (sixth nerve palsy, false localizing sign) or transient visual obscurations
- Papilledema (disk hyperemia, venous distention, swelling of optic cup with elevation of vessels, blurring of disk margin, loss of central retinal venous pulsations, hemorrhages, exudates)
- *Cushing reflex when severe:* bradycardia, systolic hypertension, and hypopnea
- *Herniation syndromes:* uncal, central (diencephalic), cerebellar tonsillar (see Chapter 17).

## Evaluation

The patient's level of consciousness should be assessed and focal abnormalities and papilledema identified. Neuroimaging, preferably with MRI, will identify structural lesions that may respond to neurosurgical treatment. Lumbar puncture should not be deferred before CT or MRI (see Chapter 2). When raised intracranial pressure is moderate or severe and is likely to persist more than 24 hours, an intracranial pressure bolt will monitor pressure continuously.

## Treatment

Several general steps are helpful in treating increased intracranial pressure:
- Elevate head and body 30° to optimize venous drainage.
- Reduce fever (increases cerebral metabolic demand and blood flow).
- Restrict fluid intake (approximately 1000 mL/24 h).
- Maintain osmolarity at 305 to 315 mOsm/L.

Specific measures include:
- *Hyperventilation* is the maneuver that most rapidly decreases intracranial pressure, diminishing cerebral blood flow and volume through vasoconstriction. After intubation, the goal is a $PCO_2$ of 25 to 30 mm Hg; $PCO_2$ below 25 mm Hg dangerously reduces cerebral blood flow. These effects last only hours and are a temporizing measure.
- *Mannitol* decreases pressure over 10 to 20 minutes; it is a hyperosmotic agent, drawing water from the brain and inducing diuresis. Initial doses are 1 to 2 g/kg for severely increased pressure, followed by 50 to 300 mg/kg every 6 hours, based on clinical status and serum osmolarity. Use is usually limited to 24 to 72 hours. Furosemide (Lasix) and glycerol serve a similar purpose.
- Corticosteroids are effective against vaso-

genic edema due to brain tumor, surgery, and radiation, but they are not effective against cytotoxic edema due to stroke or cerebral anoxia. Their mechanism of action is unknown; the onset of effect is minutes to hours after an intravenous dose. Dexamethasone (Decadron) is used most often (it has minimal mineralocorticoid effects). The initial dosage is 5 to 25 mg i.v., then 2 to 8 mg i.v. or p.o. every 6 hours, depending on severity. Corticosteroids should be given with $H_2$ blockers (ranitidine, cimetidine) to prevent GI bleeding.

- *Ventricular drainage* by a neurosurgeon effectively treats acute hydrocephalus with raised intracranial pressure, which occurs in subarachnoid hemorrhage, posterior fossa tumor, and meningitis.
- Primary disorders should be treated as soon as possible (e.g., tumor debulking, ventricular drainage of acute hydrocephalus).

*CONTROVERSY: Pentobarbital-induced coma is a controversial last resort to decrease intracranial pressure. Controlled clinical trials do not support the benefit of its routine use.*

# INTRACRANIAL HYPOTENSION

## Pathophysiology

Cerebrospinal fluid fistulas causing CSF leakage are the most common true sources of intracranial hypotension. These may result from dural tears from earlier lumbar puncture (suspect with post–lumbar puncture headache), skull fracture (leakage into the nasal passages causes CSF rhinorrhea; leakage into the external auditory canal causes CSF otorrhea), neurosurgery, skull bone tumors, severe dehydration, and ventricular shunts that are set at too low a pressure (siphon effect). Intracranial hypotension may also occur without recognizable cause.

Intracranial hypotension may be misdiagnosed if the needle incompletely penetrates the subarachnoid space and yields a falsely low pressure. Spinal subarachnoid block (e.g., spinal tumor) may also yield falsely low CSF pressures.

## Clinical Features

Postural headaches, triggered by sitting or standing and relieved by reclining, are the main symptom of intracranial hypotension. Headaches are aggravated by cough, strain, and Valsalva's maneuver. Dizziness, nausea, vomiting, and diplopia (sixth nerve palsy) may occur. The most serious complications are subdural hematoma and hygroma (a loculated CSF collection). CSF rhinorrhea may cause clear discharge from the nose or salty taste. CSF otorrhea may cause ear fullness, decreased hearing, and clear discharge from the ear canal.

## Evaluation

Postural headache and prior lumbar puncture, head injury, or neurosurgery strongly suggests the diagnosis. Patients with rhinorrhea or otorrhea should collect the discharge for analysis of transferrin or glucose (not present in normal nasal or aural discharges). Radionuclide cisternography can track CSF leaks. CT with thin cuts and "bone windows" through temporal structures can identify subtle fractures. In idiopathic cases, MRI may show meningeal enhancement.

## Treatment

Bed rest often leads to resolution of spontaneous and lumbar puncture-induced intracranial hypotension. **PEARL: For refractory post–lumbar puncture headache, an epidural blood patch (autologous blood injected near the CSF leak) is often dramatically effective; epidural saline infusion (over 48 hours) may also be effective.** Neurosurgical closure of skull defects or adjustment of shunt valve pressure may be required.

# 5
## CHAPTER

# *Neck and Back Pain*

## CLINICAL APPROACH

You will encounter patients with neck or back pain in all clinical settings—emergency room, office, or inpatient ward. Regardless of where the patient is seen, the immediate objective is to establish whether the underlying cause is serious or benign. **PEARL: Back pain associated with active systemic infection or malignancy, especially if it is associated with myelopathy on exam, is a medical emergency. Key symptoms and signs of myelopathy that should raise a red flag include bilateral leg weakness, a sensory level, and incontinence.** In patients without myelopathy, the history and physical exam are used to distinguish between disease of nerve roots (e.g., herniated disk with radiculopathy) and disease of soft tissue (e.g., muscle sprain).

Historical features of importance include the location of the pain and whether it radiates to the limbs. Try to define an inciting injury and the temporal features (i.e., a gradual versus sudden onset, and a progressive versus stable versus recurrent course). Identify exacerbants and palliants, such as position, activities (bending, straining, sneezing, exercise), time of day, heat, massage, medications, and menses. A history of systemic illness or symptoms such as fever, malaise or weight loss, diabetes, vascular disease, tuberculosis, arthritis, cancer, and medications may suggest an underlying cause. Finally, associated neurologic symptoms (e.g., weakness, sensory loss or disturbance, gait difficulty, or bowel or bladder dysfunction) help to determine the nature and urgency of the problem.

In the physical exam, search for features of infection or malignancy. Check the patient's temperature; palpate lower extremity pulses; and perform abdominal, pelvic, lymph node, and rectal exams. Identify bony tenderness, paraspinal muscle spasm, and bony curvature, and test the range of motion. The neurologic exam is critical. Define any deficits in muscle tone, bulk, or strength; look for fasciculations, reflex abnormalities or asymmetry, and areas of sensory loss.

Distinguishing between muscle weakness and limited movement secondary to pain is important but sometimes difficult. **PEARL: True weakness is constant in degree throughout the range of motion of a muscle, but pain-limited weakness allows a brief period of normal strength followed by sudden "give-way."** Observe the gait, and look for a limp, footdrop, or difficulty rising on the toes or heels. Evaluate posture. Assess the range of motion of the hips, neck, and shoulders. Test for lumbosacral nerve-root involvement by straight-leg raising: While the patient lies supine and passive, lift his or her leg until discomfort is felt (90° flexion is normal in healthy patients). Discomfort radiating down the leg suggests radicular (nerve-root) involvement. Relief of pain by flexing the knee at the limit of straight-leg raising or aggravation of pain by ankle dorsiflexion at that point also suggests radicular pathology.

# SYNDROMES

*Local back pain* is not specific for any etiology. Patients often describe steady and aching pain and can point to a specific locus. Paraspinal muscle spasm frequently accompanies local pain from any cause and often contributes to the pain.

*Radiculopathies* produce pain radiating into a limb. The pain typically fluctuates with position and activity. Coughing, straining, sneezing, and straight-leg raising may evoke radicular pain, whereas lying on the unaffected side with the painful leg flexed may relieve it. Other neurologic signs and symptoms depend on the nerve root involved (Table 5–1).

The *cauda equina syndrome* consists of paraparesis with lower extremity muscle wasting and

**Table 5–1. NEUROLOGIC DEFICITS ASSOCIATED WITH COMMON RADICULAR SYNDROMES**

| Root Level | Distribution of Sensory Loss | Motor Weakness | Reflex Loss |
|---|---|---|---|
| L4 | Anterior thigh, inner calf, foot | Knee extension | Patellar |
| L5 | Outer calf, great toe | Toe dorsiflexion | None |
| S1 | Outer calf, foot, posterior thigh | Knee flexion, foot flexion | Achilles |
| C6 | Anterior upper arm, radial forearm, thumb | Forearm flexion | Biceps or brachio-radialis |
| C7 | 2nd, 3rd fingers | Forearm extension, wrist extension, hand grip | Triceps |
| C8 | 4th, 5th fingers | Wrist flexion, intrinsic hand muscles | None |

hypotonia, leg pain and impaired sensation, and bowel and bladder dysfunction.

*Myelopathy* does not cause pain. Weakness occurs in muscle groups below the level involved and is accompanied by spasticity and increased deep tendon reflexes. Initially, this may produce only a mild gait disturbance. Because compression usually affects the posterior aspect of the cord early, posterior column vibration and position sense loss may be an early sign. A spinal sensory level and bladder and bowel dysfunction can occur. When compressive bony disease is the cause, radicular signs (as already described) may be present at the level of the compression.

## DIAGNOSTIC TESTS

*Plain films* may reveal congenital abnormalities, metabolic bone disease, and degenerative spine disease with changes in disk space height, osteophyte formation, or altered alignment. Straightening or alteration of the normal lordosis of the cervical or lumbosacral spine suggests paraspinal muscle spasm. Bony erosion may occur with metastases. Plain films do not directly assess disk herniation or show the spinal cord or nerve roots. *Bone scan* is more sensitive than plain films for diagnosing spinal metastases or infection.

*Computed tomography (CT)* scan is most useful in assessing disk disease and spinal stenosis. It provides good anatomic definition, especially of bony structures. Because of time constraints, CT is most useful to evaluate only one to three vertebral levels or when combined with myelography.

*Magnetic resonance imaging (MRI)* provides modest information about bony structures (unless marrow is involved) but is more helpful than plain films or CT to examine soft tissues and neurologic structures. It is particularly helpful for evaluating spinal abscesses or tumors and disk herniation that compromises the spinal canal. The severity of disk or bone disease on MRI may not correlate with the severity of clinical features, however. Typically, the MRI scan findings are more abnormal than the patient's actual condition. **PEARL: Only one region of the spine (cervical, thoracic, or lumbar) is studied in one MRI session.**

*Myelography* involves injection of contrast dye into the subarachnoid space. Subsequent radiographic images identify obstruction to the flow of the contrast within the thecal sac or compromise of the exiting nerve roots. CSF can be acquired at the same time; its analysis helps to diagnose infection, malignancy, or inflammatory disease. Postmyelographic CT imaging provides better anatomic definition than CT alone and may identify smaller lesions.

*Electromyography* can reveal physiologic dysfunction, rather than the anatomic abnormalities revealed by the other tests. Evidence of denervation (sharp waves and fibrillation potentials) in the distribution of a nerve root may suggest radicular injury, but a delay of several weeks from the onset of nerve-root injury is necessary for such findings to develop.

## SPECIFIC DISORDERS

### Strain

**Lumbosacral and cervical strains** are self-limited injuries resulting from minor traumas (e.g., lifting, falls, or "whiplash") that affect muscles and ligaments, not bones or disks. The symptoms of a strain may occur together with those of disk herniation and degenerative spine disease. Diagnosis is clinical, relying on historical features of the injury, findings of localized pain with or without muscle spasm, absence of neurologic signs or symptoms, normal x-rays, and response to conservative treatment.

## Disk Herniation

Disk herniation most commonly occurs in the cervical or lumbar spines of adults. Disk herniation often results from a flexion injury, from either a single trauma or recurrent injuries such as repeated bending and lifting. Often no precipitant is identified. The annulus fibrosus allows the nucleus pulposus to prolapse, sometimes protruding through the annulus or extruding as a free fragment within the spinal canal. The pain usually begins acutely and may be severe; often any movement aggravates it. Focal tenderness may be present.

In the lumbar spine, disks usually herniate laterally, compressing the nerve root against the lamina and producing local pain and radicular syndromes at the affected level. The L4-5 and L5-S1 disk spaces are most commonly affected. Cervical disk herniation most commonly involves the C5-6 and C6-7 disk spaces. Disk herniation in the neck usually occurs in the weaker, midline portion of the posterior longitudinal ligament, producing a myelopathy often accompanied by a radiculopathy.

## Degenerative Disease

Degenerative disease of the spine occurs with aging, producing **spondylosis**—bony overgrowth that may be hastened by recurrent or chronic trauma. It is most common in the cervical and lumbar spine. **PEARL: Radiographic evidence of**

**spondylosis is very common, occurring in three-fourths of asymptomatic patients over age 70.**

With age, the water content of the vertebral disk declines, so the disk thins and becomes more fragile and often bulges posteriorly. Spinal ligaments and the annulus fibrosus also progressively weaken and calcify. Hypertrophic changes occur at the margins of the vertebral bodies and at the facet joints, producing bone spurs and osteophytes. Osteoporosis can contribute to vertebral flattening or collapse. Intervertebral joints may become subluxed, further compromising the spinal canal and intervertebral foramina.

Spondylosis is distinguished clinically from disk herniation by the chronic, progressive nature of the symptoms, but they commonly co-exist. Compromise of intervertebral foramina or the spinal canal may occur with either disorder. In the cervical spine, myelopathic and radiculopathic features often co-exist, with prominent local pain and restricted lateral flexion and rotation of the neck. In the lumbosacral spine, radicular symptoms predominate.

## Tumors

Metastatic disease is the most common malignancy affecting the spine. Spinal metastases often originate in breast, lung, and prostate cancers and less commonly in thyroid, kidney, stomach, and uterine cancers, as well as multiple myeloma and lymphoma. Pain generally begins insidiously but is unremitting and progressive. Back pain unrelieved by lying down suggests an intrathecal mass, such as metastasis. Focal tenderness is commonly found and has localizing value.

Cord compression with myelopathy frequently complicates metastatic disease because of vertebral body collapse or intradural or extradural metastatic deposits. Myelopathic signs call for emergent radiation or surgical treatment to avoid impending paraplegia and incontinence, which may develop precipitously and irreversibly. In this setting, steroids (25 mg of i.v. dexamethasone, followed by 4 mg every 6 hours, orally or intravenously) are given emergently to reduce edema.

## Infectious Diseases

Infectious diseases of the spine include *vertebral osteomyelitis*, which generally arises by hematogenous spread from a primary site elsewhere. This produces severe back pain with localized tenderness, often with fever and malaise. The white blood cell count and sedimentation rate are usually elevated. *Epidural abscess* may follow from vertebral osteomyelitis or occur independently. Neurologic signs of cord compression follow the onset of back pain after a variable period and may progress rapidly, requiring emergent neuroimaging and surgical drainage of the abscess. Surgical drainage of an epidural abscess is followed by treatment with parenteral antibiotics for 3 to 4 weeks, or up to 6 to 8 weeks if vertebral osteomyelitis is also present.

## TREATMENT

Treatments specific to disorders such as malignancy and infection have already been discussed. When these diagnoses are suspected, urgent neuroimaging and intervention are required. General approaches to treatment for other types of low back and neck pain follow.

*Conservative nonsurgical therapies* are graded to the severity and acuity of symptoms. **PEARL: Patients with mild or chronic symptoms should be instructed in proper posture, particularly when bend-**

**ing or lifting.** Activities that incite pain should be avoided. Ice is recommended in the acute phase; after that, local heat may relieve symptoms. Analgesics, particularly nonsteroidal anti-inflammatory agents, are helpful. Physical therapy during nonacute phases, to strengthen the major back muscles and improve posture, may help to prevent recurrent injury. Overweight patients should be urged to lose weight. When patients present with acute, severe low back or neck pain, strict rest on a firm bed was often recommended but is no more helpful than usual activity, according to current literature. Acute neck pain may respond to a cervical soft collar or traction.

Analgesics and anti-inflammatory agents (including steroids) may be supplemented with antispasmodic agents or muscle relaxors such as diazepam or cyclobenzaprine hydrochloride. These agents are most effective when used for a limited period. Opioids are best avoided except to treat acute, severe pain. Reintroduction of full activity after a few days or weeks of limited activity should begin slowly after symptoms have remitted.

*Surgical treatment* is reserved for patients who have failed conservative therapy, or who display acute, objective signs of radiculopathy or myelopathy. Evidence of a new cauda equina syndrome or an acute progressive myelopathy calls for emergent surgery. **PEARL: Elective surgery depends on the clinical condition of the patient; radiographic indications for surgery (except for neoplastic or infectious disease) do not exist.** Although the anterior-posterior diameter of the cervical spinal canal is said to be inadequate if it measures less than 9 to 10 mm, the degree of narrowing may not correlate with the *clinical* deficit or prognosis. Surgical decompression in such patients may improve the neurologic deficit but is more effective in preventing progression. Chronic pain syndromes respond poorly to surgical treatment and are often associated with psychiatric comorbidity.

# 6
## CHAPTER

# *Dizziness and Imbalance*

Dizziness and imbalance are common complaints in neurologic practice. **Dizziness** refers to a subjective perception, whereas **imbalance** is the physical manifestation of altered equilibrium in three-dimensional space. Like the word "confusion," "dizziness" is a confusing term that must *always* be qualified further. Dizziness and imbalance usually arise from disturbances in central or peripheral vestibular pathways, proprioceptive pathways, or the cerebellum.

Reports of dizziness increase with aging. It is among the most frequent symptoms reported by persons over age 75 and often goes undiagnosed and untreated. A major consequence of dizziness is falls, resulting in head trauma, hip fracture, and death.

## CLINICAL CATEGORIES OF DIZZINESS

Four clinical categories of dizziness are recognized; make every effort to pigeonhole the patient's report into one of these categories:

# Vertigo

**Vertigo** is the perception that one's self or the environment is moving. The perceived movement is usually rotatory, with a spinning sensation, but it may be translational, reported as swaying back and forth or a sense of falling. Accompanying symptoms are nausea, vomiting, staggering gait, diaphoresis, and dysphoria. **Impulsion,** a feeling that the body is being hurled or pulled in space, may be reported. **Oscillopsia** is the visual illusion of the environment moving back and forth.

With active vertigo, **nystagmus** (involuntary, rhythmic movement of the eyeball) should be demonstrable. Nystagmus is the extraocular correlate of active vertigo. The slow phase of nystagmus usually points toward the abnormal labyrinth. The patient perceives falling to the side of the slow phase or abnormal labyrinth. *Vertical nystagmus* during either upgaze or downgaze implies a central vestibular disturbance.

Vertigo implicates a disturbance in the peripheral labyrinth, vestibular division of the eighth cranial nerve, and the brainstem vestibular nuclei with their connections to the cerebellum, oculomotor nuclei, reticular activating system, and the spinal cord (Table 6–1). Rarely, vertigo may be of cortical origin, associated with complex partial seizures.

# Presyncope

**Presyncope** refers to a sense of impending fainting or loss of consciousness and is often described as faintness, lightheadedness, wooziness,

### Table 6–1. COMMON CAUSES OF VERTIGO

Acute peripheral vestibulopathy (vestibular neuronitis)
Acute labyrinthitis
Benign positional vertigo
Ménière's disease
Post-traumatic vertigo
Vertebrobasilar insufficiency
Posterior fossa tumors
Multiple sclerosis
Physiologic causes (motion sickness, fear of heights)
Familial episodic ataxia

or giddiness. Sweating, nausea, pallor, and telescoping of peripheral vision often accompany it. Vertigo is absent. There may be transient loss of consciousness, a symptom not seen with vestibular dysfunction. **PEARL: Presyncope implicates a disturbance in either the *quantity* of cerebral blood flow or its *quality* (e.g., hypoxia, hypoglycemia).** Disturbances in cardiac output and impaired vasomotor reflexes are the usual culprits (Table 6–2).

The history should focus on episodes provoked with positional change, cardiac disease, and situations that promote dehydration and autonomic dysfunction. Other clues are a recent, prolonged episode of bed rest, which typically exacerbates orthostatic hypotension. The patient should be examined for orthostatic vital signs, as well as stigmata of cardiac disease. Confirmatory diagnostic tests include electrocardiography, Holter monitoring, and echocardiography.

## Disequilibrium

**Disequilibrium** refers to perceived imbalance while standing or walking. Somatic or visual

**Table 6–2. COMMON CAUSES
OF PRESYNCOPE**

Vasovagal syncope (emotional reflex)

Orthostatic hypotension
  Volume depletion
  Drug-related effects
  Peripheral neuropathy
  Central autonomic insufficiency (Parkinson's disease, Shy-
    Drager syndrome)

Micturition syncope

Strenuous coughing

Cardiac arrhythmia

Aortic stenosis

Mitral stenosis

Hypertrophic cardiomyopathy

Carotid sinus hypersensitivity (rare)

Vertebrobasilar insufficiency (rare)

*sensory deprivation* or *loss* may lead to imbalance and incoordination. The patient often reports walking "like a drunken sailor." Complaints of vertigo are absent. Peripheral neuropathy, posterior column dysfunction, cerebellar disease, and impaired central integration of visual, proprioceptive, and cerebellar information are common sources (Table 6–3). Physical exam identifies stigmata of the primary disorder, such as impaired vision, proprioceptive loss, rigidity, tremor, poor postural reflexes, or cerebellar ataxia with a wide-based reeling gait. Very often, the "central integration program" for integrating these inputs with dynamic motor output is defective. Persons with visual field deficits also have much trouble navigating in space. Disequilibrium and imbalance (discussed later) overlap.

### Table 6–3. COMMON CAUSES OF
### DISEQUILIBRIUM AND IMBALANCE

Cerebellar dysfunction
  Cerebellar hemorrhage and infarction
  Wernicke's encephalopathy
  Alcoholic cerebellar degeneration
  Drug-induced cerebellar degeneration
  Hypothyroidism
  Paraneoplastic cerebellar degeneration
  Idiopathic or heredofamilial spinocerebellar degeneration

Extrapyramidal dysfunction

Sensory ataxias

Posterior column–large-fiber dysfunction
  Diabetic polyneuropathy
  Toxins, alcohol, and prescription medicine
  Tabes dorsalis
  HIV myelopathy
  Vitamin $B_{12}$ deficiency
  Antiretroviral agents

Cerebral dysfunction
  Infarction

Multiple sclerosis

Drugs
  Alcohol
  Sedatives (benzodiazepines and barbiturates)
  Anticonvulsants
  Neuroleptics
  Antiarrhythmics
  Quinine and quinidine
  Salicylates
  Antibiotics (including antiretrovirals)
  Chemotherapy agents

Posterior fossa tumors

Vertebrobasilar insufficiency

Multiple sensory impairments

## Psychogenic Dizziness

**Psychogenic dizziness** is invoked when complaints cannot be readily classified into one of the above categories. Patients report symptoms of "swimming in the head," giddiness, wooziness, and confusion. They often have chronic hyperventilation, anxiety, depression, or other nonspecific emotional or mental aberrations or are experiencing subtle impairment of neuropsychological function by recreational or prescription drugs (Table 6–4). Inquire about psychiatric history, situations that precipitate the symptoms, and whether hyperventilation, paresthesias of the limbs, and panic are associated with the attack.

An exam of these patients is typically normal. Hyperventilation for 3 minutes may reproduce the attack. In contrast to the other categories just described, symptoms are often continuous rather than episodic (although hyperventilation and panic attacks are episodic), and there are no associated focal neurologic symptoms or exam abnormalities. Treatment involves reassurance and treatment of any primary psychiatric disorder.

## CLINICAL EVALUATION OF THE "DIZZY" PATIENT

It is crucial to ask, "Can you describe what you mean by feeling dizzy?" The sensation of *spinning*

### Table 6–4. COMMON CAUSES OF PSYCHOGENIC DIZZINESS

Hyperventilation syndrome

Anxiety

Depression

Somatization

Panic disorder

Substance abuse

Other nonspecific causes

implicates the vestibular system. Sensations of *imbalance* suggest central nervous system (CNS) involvement. Peripheral vertigo is rarely persistent, but chronic dizziness suggests a central or psychogenic cause. Central causes of dizziness are usually less affected by head movement or positional changes; orthostatic hypotension, on the other hand, causes dizziness on rising from sitting or lying positions. Peripheral vertigo will be associated with a veering gait and unsteady stance along with severe nausea, perspiration, and tachycardia. Cochlear symptoms, such as hearing impairment or tinnitus, imply a peripheral lesion affecting both divisions of the eighth nerve or the cochlea and labyrinth. Recent head trauma may cause labyrinthine and central integration disturbances. Vertigo precipitated by Valsalva's maneuver or sneezing suggests a perilymphatic fistula. The presence of other neurologic symptoms—visual changes, paralysis, altered consciousness, headaches, binocular diplopia, or frank blindness—implicates brainstem or cerebral causes. Leg numbness is frequent when peripheral neuropathy or proprioceptive dysfunction are a cause of disequilibrium. Cardiac symptoms and a family history of dizziness or hearing loss should be documented.

Table 6–5 lists the areas of special focus during the neurologic exam of the dizzy patient. An important localizing finding of the neurologic examination is nystagmus. With dysfunction of one labyrinth, there is a slow phase of eye deviation toward the abnormal labyrinth, followed by a fast cortical corrective movement (nystagmus) in the opposite direction. Nystagmus is named for the direction of its fast phase. With peripheral vestibular disorders, the slow phase is unidirectional and directed at the abnormal ear, with the fast phase away. The corrective nystagmus is rotatory or horizontal and always unidirectional. The patient feels that he or she is falling to the side of the abnormal

**Table 6–5. FEATURES TO HIGHLIGHT
DURING NEUROLOGIC EXAM
OF THE "DIZZY" PATIENT**

---

Extraocular movements (vertical nystagmus suggests
  brainstem dysfunction)

Weber's and Rinne's tests

Whisper

Vibration and joint-position sense

Past pointing (patient stands and does finger-nose-finger with
  eyes open and closed; misses the target with cerebellar-
  vestibular disorders)

Tandem gait and Romberg testing

Passive and active rotational tests (patient sits on stool that
  can be actively or passively rotated with eyes open, then
  closed)

---

ear or toward the slow phase. With CNS disorders,
the nystagmus is multidirectional or vertical.

In addition, a "dizziness simulation battery" can
be performed, using equipment readily available on
the ward and in the clinic setting (Table 6–6). Maneuvers that reproduce the patient's symptoms ex-
actly give insight into the cause of the dizziness syndrome and point to further avenues of investigation.

## LABORATORY TESTING

Medical evaluation of the dizzy patient may
include electrocardiography, echocardiography,
and Holter monitoring. Venereal Disease Research Laboratory (VDRL) and thyroid function
testing should be considered in those with chronic
vertigo. Neurodiagnostic testing might involve an
audiologic evaluation with attention to air and
bone conduction. Caloric tests assess the periph-

**Table 6–6. THE "DIZZINESS SIMULATION BATTERY"**

Orthostatic signs while lying, sitting, and standing for 3 min (useful for those on multiple-drug regimens)

Valsalva's maneuver

Forced hyperventilation for 3 min

Nylen-Bárány maneuvers (useful in benign positional vertigo)

Carotid sinus massage

Sudden turns while walking

eral vestibular apparatus, and may induce vomiting. The **brainstem auditory evoked potential (BAEP)** tests the integrity of the eighth nerve and brainstem pathways from the cochlea to the auditory cortex. In some cases of subtle vestibular dysfunction, electronystagmography determines any directional preponderance of evoked nystagmus and canal paresis; this test is helpful in separating central versus peripheral causes of vertigo.

Computed tomography (CT) of the brain and skull is particularly useful in demonstrating lesions in sinus anatomy. Magnetic resonance imaging (MRI) is clearly the most useful test for investigating dizziness ascribed to brainstem lesions, multiple sclerosis, and craniovertebral junction abnormalities.

## COMMON ENTITIES CAUSING DIZZINESS

### Benign Positional Vertigo

This syndrome is common in older persons. Spinning dizziness occurs when reclining at night, turning over in bed, rising in the morning, or turning the head rapidly. **PEARL: The distinction between benign positional vertigo (BPV) and other vestibular disorders is that although all have a positional *exacerbation* of symptoms, assuming a particular position *produces* symptoms in this disorder.** Usually one or two characteristic movements elicit symptoms. Hearing is intact. The Nylen-Bárány maneuver, a simple office screening test, reproduces symptoms: There is a latency of several seconds before vertigo and nystagmus appear, their duration is brief, and repetitive maneuvers gradually extinguish the vertigo and nystagmus. BPV may be precipitated by prior middle ear infections or head trauma.

Abnormal function of the otoliths in the semicircular canals is believed to cause most cases. Age-related degenerative changes in the vestibular apparatus account for the increased prevalence with aging. Symptoms tend to last days to weeks; recurrent attacks are not uncommon. Although medications such as meclizine are commonly prescribed, they are not specific. A soft cervical collar may lessen neck motion. Labyrinthine exercises prescribed by specialized therapists can accelerate recovery.

## Motion Sickness

Some persons are constitutionally prone to vertigo, nausea, and diaphoresis when a mismatch between visual, proprioceptive, and vestibular input occurs. The usual precipitants are automobile and ship travel, coupled with the inability to fixate on an outside reference and thus suppress the vestibulo-ocular reflex.

## Acute Labyrinthitis (Vestibular Neuronitis)

This syndrome usually follows a prior upper respiratory infection and is characterized by rapid onset of vertigo, severe nausea, retching, and nystagmus. Patients may complain of tinnitus and ear fullness, but hearing is usually normal. Caloric testing demonstrates canal paresis on the involved side, without evoked nystagmus. This disorder is generally self-limited, lasting days to weeks, and rarely produces permanent symptoms, but it may recur. Severe episodes require acute treatment with intravenous diazepam and fluid repletion. Bed rest and gaze fixation minimize discomfort.

## Ménière's Disease

Attributed to idiopathic dilatation of the endolymphatic system (endolymphatic hydrops), this entity is typified by recurrent attacks of roaring tinnitus, low-frequency hearing loss, ear fullness, and intense vertigo. There may be chronic imbalance between attacks. The age at onset is usually in the fourth through sixth decades and the syndrome is rare after age 70. Hearing loss is unilateral and sensorineural in nature and may become progressive with permanent tinnitus. MRI will exclude a cerebellopontine angle tumor, and lab testing will exclude infection or stasis in the labyrinth (e.g., syphilis, hyperlipidemia). Therapy includes a low-salt diet, diuretics, antihistamines, and (in disabling, refractory cases) selective surgical obliteration of the labyrinth or eighth nerve.

## Postconcussive Syndrome

Following head injury, many patients experience a self-limited, transient syndrome of headache, presyncopal sensations, positional vertigo, impaired concentration, and emotionality. When there is associated labyrinthine concussion, gas-

trointestinal symptoms, nystagmus, and falling to
the side of the affected ear are also typical. Therapy is symptomatic, and the disorder improves
over several days to weeks. Trauma sufficient to
produce a perilymphatic fistula may result in a
chronic or recurrent syndrome. These patients
may have recurrent vertigo and conductive hearing loss. The fistula usually heals spontaneously,
but surgical correction may be required.

## Vertebrobasilar Insufficiency

**PEARL: Although vertigo is the most common
symptom of vertebrobasilar insufficiency, vertigo
alone should not be accepted as diagnostic of this entity.** The patient must be asked about other posterior circulation symptoms: diplopia, tinnitus, peri-
oral numbness, dysarthria, dysphagia, occipital
headache, ataxia, visual field deficits, and motor
and sensory abnormalities occurring bilaterally.
In addition to signs of brainstem dysfunction, nystagmus will be multidirectional or vertical. Evaluation includes MRI (better visualization of brain
stem and cerebellar structures than with CT),
Doppler ultrasound, transcranial Doppler, and
transesophageal echocardiography.

Some persons with severe cervical spondylosis
develop neurovascular compression of the vertebral arteries. Symptoms are precipitated by head
extension. Evaluation includes cervical spine films.
In addition, transcranial Doppler studies sometimes demonstrate reversible disruptions in vertebrobasilar flow with specific head maneuvers.

## Central Vertigo

Typical causes of central vertigo are demyelinating disease and brainstem or cerebellar in-

farction. Although clinically similar to peripheral causes of vertigo, central vertigo is usually less intense. The Nylen-Bárány maneuvers demonstrate a more immediate onset of sustained nystagmus that is less amenable to extinction.

## Orthostatic Hypotension

Drugs that commonly cause postural (orthostatic) hypotension include antihypertensives, levodopa, neuroleptics, and tricyclic antidepressants.

## Vasodepressor Syncope

Fear, anxiety, or pain usually precedes simple fainting. There is associated weakness, epigastric distress, perspiration, restlessness, and pallor. Consciousness is restored rapidly with recumbence, but there may be a few myoclonic jerks when hypotension is prolonged.

## Multiple Sensory Impairment

**PEARL: Multiple sensory impairment is a common and underdiagnosed cause of gait unsteadiness in elderly persons.** The additive effects of impaired visual acuity due to cataracts, impaired proprioception from mild peripheral sensory neuropathy due to degeneration of large-fiber sensory neurons, and superimposed mild cerebellar dysfunction all contribute. Some elderly persons are prone to "drop attacks," sudden loss of postural tone with falling without loss of consciousness. Persons with Parkinson's disease or cerebellar dysfunction often report unsteadiness. The physical exam will demonstrate impaired vision, proprioceptive loss, postural instability, and an ataxic gait.

## Vertebrobasilar Migraine

This relatively rare variant of migraine usually affects adolescent women. Signs and symptoms are similar to those of vertebrobasilar insufficiency associated with a severe migrainous occipital headache. The initial episode will require investigation by MRI and vascular ultrasound.

## Miscellaneous Entities

Other CNS disorders that produce vertigo include multiple sclerosis, migraine, and rarely seizures. In addition, some medications may induce vertigo, dysarthria, and incoordination. Common culprits include salicylates, benzodiazepines, anticonvulsants, alcohol, antibiotics, and chemotherapeutic agents.

## TREATMENT OF DIZZINESS

Benzodiazepines and beta-blockers are specific treatments for dizziness that is caused by hyperventilation. Nonspecific treatments for vertigo include:

- Meclizine 12.5 to 25 mg p.o. every 6 hours
- Dimenhydrinate 25 to 50 mg p.o. every 6 hours
- Scopolamine 0.5 mg transdermally every 72 hours
- Diazepam 2 to 4 mg p.o. tid
- Prochlorperazine (Compazine) 25 to 50 mg p.o. every 6 hours

Adverse effects of these medicines include sedation, dry mouth, and blurred vision. Scopolamine may cause confusion, urinary retention, and constipation in the elderly.

For patients with chronic or recurrent vertigo, consider a course of promethazine (Phenergan) plus ephedrine. This combination has been shown to reduce vestibular firing; ephedrine counteracts the drowsiness induced by phenergan. Around-the-clock meclizine is an alternative. Labyrinthine exercises by trained therapists may improve benign positional vertigo.

# CAUSES OF PREDOMINANT IMBALANCE

## Sensory Ataxias

Sensory ataxia results from impaired proprioception, usually at the level of the peripheral nerves, posterior columns in the cord, or sensory centers in the brain. Clinical findings include impaired vibration and joint position, a "stamp and strike" gait, and a positive Romberg test. Commonly encountered clinical entities include:

- Diabetic polyneuropathy
- Large-fiber neuropathy from toxins, alcohol, and prescription medicine
  - Cisplatin
  - Isoniazid
  - Pyridoxine excess
- Tabes dorsalis
- Human immunodeficiency virus (HIV) vacuolar myelopathy
- Multiple sclerosis
- Vitamin $B_{12}$ deficiency
- Hypothyroidism
- Antiretroviral agents

## Cerebellar Ataxias

**Alcoholic cerebellar degeneration** occurs in chronic alcoholics and is usually associated with other neurologic or medical complications of chronic drinking. It consists of a gradually progressive gait ataxia, mainly in the lower limbs. MRI demonstrates midline cerebellar atrophy. With adequate nutrition and abstinence from alcohol, the condition can stabilize.

Chronic use of *phenytoin* has been associated with a pancerebellar syndrome consisting of nystagmus, dysarthria, and limb and trunk ataxia. Drug levels of phenytoin have often been in the toxic range.

*Hypothyroidism* can affect all levels of the neuraxis, and cerebellar dysfunction is common, usually manifest as a gait ataxia. Patients nearly always have the physical stigmata of hypothyroidism.

*Cerebellar infarctions and hemorrhages* are usually associated with underlying hypertension. The presentation may be subtle, with occipital headache and mild ataxia. Patients complaining of headache and a rapidly declining level of consciousness should be forced to walk so that truncal ataxia can be assessed. CT is usually adequate for diagnosis. Cerebellar vascular disease is the one cerebrovascular lesion in which acute neurosurgical intervention may be lifesaving.

## Cerebellopontine-Angle Tumors

These tumors are typically schwannomas or meningiomas and most commonly present with progressive unilateral hearing loss for high frequencies; poor word recognition is characteristic. Vertigo, tinnitus, and fifth and seventh cranial nerve dysfunction are unusual accompaniments.

As cerebellar and brainstem compression ensues, gait ataxia may develop. The neurologic exam will show impaired hearing, impaired corneal sensation, facial weakness, unilateral dysmetria, gait ataxia, and rarely nystagmus. MRI is the imaging procedure of choice. BAEPs may demonstrate slowing of wave I. All adults with acquired sensorineural hearing loss should undergo MRI to rule out a cerebellopontine-angle tumor. Surgical therapy is usually recommended.

## Posterior Fossa Tumors

These mass lesions commonly present with occipital headache, ataxia, nausea, vomiting, vertigo, cranial nerve palsies, and hydrocephalus. MRI is clearly the most useful imaging modality for lesions in this region. **PEARL: If clinical symptoms and signs are worsening rapidly, a plain CT (more readily and rapidly available) may be used to screen for gross hemorrhage, edema, and hydrocephalus.** In order of frequency, the most common posterior fossa tumors are metastases, cerebellar astrocytomas, medulloblastomas, and others such as schwannomas, meningiomas, and ependymomas.

## Posterior Fossa Malformations

Arnold-Chiari malformation type 1 consists of downward displacement of the cerebellar tonsils through the foramen magnum. It presents in adulthood with occipital headaches, lower cranial nerve palsies, and gait ataxia. Hydrocephalus may occur, with nausea and vomiting. Sagittal MRI of the craniovertebral junction confirms the diagnosis. High cervical laminectomy with decompression of the posterior fossa is curative.

## Familial Episodic Ataxia

This entity is characterized by brief attacks of vertigo and slowly progressive truncal ataxia. Some cases respond to acetazolamide, a carbonic anhydrase inhibitor.

## Medications

Many medicines commonly produce imbalance and incoordination. Patients experience vertigo and, in cases of salicylate or aminoglycoside intoxication, tinnitus and hearing loss. The exam shows multidirectional nystagmus, as well as ataxia and even dysarthria if the intoxication is severe. Drug levels can document the presence of the offending agent, which typically may be alcohol, anticonvulsants, salicylates, benzodiazepines, and aminoglycosides. Treatment is discontinuation of the drug. Most of these disorders are reversible, but aminoglycoside-related ototoxicity and vestibulotoxicity may be permanent.

# 7
## CHAPTER

# *Sensory Symptoms*

You will encounter sensory symptoms in both acutely and chronically ill neurology patients. Sensory symptoms manifest as numbness, tingling, or pain. Pain is covered in other chapters. **PEARL: Be wary about complaints of "numbness," because patients who are weak without sensory changes often complain that their limbs are "numb" or "dead."**

The history and physical exam must establish the pattern of symptoms by anatomic region as well as by their onset, course, and associated features. Table 7–1 describes the common patterns of sensory deficit found in neurology patients. Patients with sensory symptoms typically suffer from stroke, degenerative spine disease, neuropathy, demyelinating disorders, and conversion disorders. Stroke is discussed in Chapter 19. Degenerative spine disease is reviewed in Chapter 5. Multiple sclerosis, the best-known demyelinating disease, is discussed in Chapter 11, and conversion disorders are covered in Chapter 13.

## MONONEUROPATHIES

**Mononeuropathies** involve one large nerve, such as a cranial nerve or the median nerve. Along with sensory complaints, pain is common.

### Table 7–1. TYPICAL PATTERNS OF SENSORY LOSS FOR NEUROLOGIC DISORDERS

| Pattern of Sensory Loss | Localization | Diagnosis (Example) |
|---|---|---|
| Palmar hand, palmar digits one to three | Single-nerve territory | Carpal tunnel syndrome |
| **"Glove and stocking":** below elbows and below knees, bilaterally, circumferentially around limbs | Multiple nerves or polyneuropathy | Diabetic neuropathy |
| No sensation below the umbilicus | Spinal cord | Metastatic cord compression |
| No sensation of trunk from nipples to umbilicus, but normal above and below this area | Central spinal cord | Syrinx |
| Hemibody loss, including the trunk and face | Thalamus | Stroke |
| Distal arm and leg on one side | Cortex | Stroke |

**Compression neuropathy,** the most common cause of mononeuropathy, results from external or internal pressure along any point of the course of a nerve. **Entrapment neuropathy** is a form of compression neuropathy due to constricting pressure when a nerve lies in a narrow anatomic passage.

**Carpal tunnel syndrome** is the most common entrapment neuropathy. Inquire about hand pain and tingling in the median nerve distribution, often at night or after vigorous activity. Symptoms often progress up the arm. Causes include overuse of the hands, particularly in occupations that involve typing or use of vibrating machinery, as well as pregnancy, rheumatoid arthritis, diabetes mellitus, acromegaly, amyloidosis, and paraproteinemia. The diagnosis is made clinically and by slowed nerve conduction velocity (NCV) across the carpal tunnel, or by an electromyography (EMG) finding of denervation of the abductor pollicis brevis (supplied by the distal median nerve). Underlying disorders such as diabetes and hypothyroidism precipitating carpal tunnel syndrome should be excluded. Patients with mild, typically sensory symptoms and NCV or EMG abnormalities may be treated with splinting or steroid injection of the carpal tunnel. Patients with more severe abnormalities and persistent complaints unresponsive to conservative measures require surgical release of the carpal tunnel.

**Ulnar nerve entrapment** at the elbow produces pain radiating distally from the elbow, associated with numbness and tingling of the ulnar fingers and palm. Loss of hand motor function and atrophy occur in more advanced cases. Elbow trauma or excessive elbow flexion may be the cause. Entrapment at the ulnar groove or cubital tunnel can be cured with surgical decompression.

**Meralgia paresthetica** is compression of the lateral femoral cutaneous nerve of the thigh as it exits the inguinal ligament. It produces tingling, pain, and numbness of the anterolateral thigh, with or without sensory impairment. Possible causes include obesity, pregnancy, recently developed ascites, or garments that compress the nerve. Relief often comes from reversing the precipitating factors, or the nerve may be injected with steroids.

**Mononeuropathy multiplex** involves multiple peripheral nerves. The causes include diabetes mellitus, sarcoidosis, vasculitis, gammopathy, and human immunodeficiency virus (HIV) infection. The distribution of the deficit is detected clinically and may be confirmed by EMG and NCV testing. Diabetes can be diagnosed with clinical and laboratory data, sarcoidosis and vasculitis can be confirmed by nerve biopsy, gammopathy is identified by serum protein electrophoresis (SPEP), and HIV infection is confirmed by antibody testing. Treatment is directed at the primary disorder.

## POLYNEUROPATHIES

**Polyneuropathy** reflects impaired sensory and motor function of many peripheral nerves. The impairment is usually symmetrical and distal more than proximal. Polyneuropathy can affect small nerves (pain, temperature, autonomic functions), large nerves (joint position sensation, tactile discrimination), or both. Diminished or absent deep tendon reflexes are seen with large-fiber neuropathies.

The causes are many: diabetes mellitus; renal failure; vitamin deficiency; connective tissue disease; cancer; gammopathy; heavy metal poisoning; and drugs such as cisplatin, vincristine, isoniazid, phenytoin, gold, and hydralazine. The clinical history and exam and classification by NCV as axonal neuropathy (normal nerve conduction) or demyelinating neuropathy (slow conduction) are helpful for diagnosis. For example, neuropathy due to gammopathy is typically demyelinating, but neuropathy due to renal failure is axonal. Neuropathy due to *diabetes mellitus,* the most common cause of chronic neuropathy, typically produces a sensory impairment or both sensory and motor impairment and is often painful. In many patients, the cause of neuropathy is unknown.

**PEARL: Patients with polyneuropathy will need treatment of the primary disease, as well as physical therapy and assistive devices.**

*Nutritional causes* of chronic neuropathy include thiamine deficiency in alcoholics, $B_{12}$ deficiency in pernicious anemia, pyridoxine deficiency in patients taking isoniazid for tuberculosis, and folic acid deficiency in patients taking phenytoin or phenobarbital. All these deficiencies may be associated with a painful sensory neuropathy. Vitamin replacement is the cornerstone of therapy.

*Toxic causes* of neuropathy include lead, which has sensorimotor effects. Lead levels confirm the diagnosis. Patients are treated with ethylenediaminetetra-acetic acid and penicillamine after toxic exposure is terminated. Many drugs also cause neuropathy. These patients are treated by reduction of exposure and supportive therapy.

Monoclonal **gammopathy** can cause a severe, progressive, demyelinating sensorimotor neuropathy. A monoclonal spike is detected on SPEP. The primary disease may be myeloma or macroglobulinemia, but some cases are idiopathic. Neuropathy associated with gammopathy may be treated with plasmapheresis or immune globulin.

In *HIV infection*, distal sensorimotor neuropathy is often painful, predominantly sensory, and associated with loss of reflexes. Diagnosis is made clinically and confirmed by HIV testing. Tricyclic antidepressants or antiepileptic drugs reduce pain.

Sensory symptoms may appear early in the course of *multiple sclerosis*. Chapter 11 covers this disease in more detail.

**Conversion disorder** is characterized by symptoms or deficits that suggest neurologic or medical disorders but actually result from psychological factors. Diagnosis is often difficult. **Malingering** is the intentional production or exaggeration of physical or mental symptoms for personal benefit. See Chapter 13 for a fuller discussion of these topics.

# 8
## CHAPTER

# *Dementia*

**Dementia** is an acquired, persistent, usually progressive decline of intellectual function severe enough to impair social or occupational pursuits. Cardinal features are intact arousal with impairments of memory, intellect, and personality. With increased life expectancy, the incidence and prevalence of dementia are rising, imposing significant burdens on health-care services.

Dementia is distinguished from *developmental disability* because it is an *acquired* loss of normal intellect. Dementia is progressive, whereas developmental disability is static. The developmentally disabled learn and develop more slowly and to a more limited extent. Hallmarks of developmental disability include delayed developmental milestones, motor impairments (hemiplegia, diplegia, choreoathetosis), epilepsy, and behavior problems.

## FEATURES OF DEMENTIA

Short-term memory impairment is the most common and pervasive presenting feature of dementia. Higher cognitive functions may be impaired, with aphasia, apraxia, and agnosia. Patients may become easily lost or wander and may have difficulty with learned tasks such as dressing or cooking. Emotional lability or flattened affect is common. Patients often lose insight and judgment. Dementias are termed **subcortical** if there are prominent features of **bradyphrenia** (slowed thinking), forgetfulness, depressed mood, and apathy. Parkinson's disease and Huntington's disease are examples of *subcortical dementias.* In contrast, Alzheimer's and Pick's diseases are regarded as **cortical dementias** if higher cortical dysfunctions (aphasia, apraxia, agnosia) and amnesia are present.

Examining the patient for dementia includes observations of memory, thinking, concentration, attention, judgment, insight, and behavior. Bedside tests such as the Folstein Mini-Mental State Examination help to screen patients for dementia; a score below 26 (of 30) is considered abnormal. Neuropsychologic testing profiles the nature and extent of impairment and helps to track the tempo of progression. Psychiatric evaluation helps to diagnose associated depression and behavioral disturbances.

## CAUSES OF DEMENTIA

The most common causes of dementia are shown in Table 8–1.

## WORK-UP

**PEARL: There is no standard "work-up" for dementia, although certain tests should be completed**

**Table 8–1. COMMON CAUSES
OF DEMENTIA**

Alzheimer's disease (AD)

Multi-infarct (vascular) dementia

Mixed Alzheimer's and vascular dementia

Parkinson's disease

Lewy-body dementia

Cerebral tumors
   Primary (meningioma, glioma)
   Metastatic

Chronic subdural hematoma

Chronic hydrocephalus

Multiple sclerosis

Huntington's chorea (Huntington's disease)

Head trauma

Intracranial hemorrhage

CNS infections
   HIV encephalitis
   Meningitis
   Encephalitis (herpes)
   Creutzfeldt-Jakob disease
   Abscess

CNS anoxia (drug overdose, cardiac arrest)

Alcohol and other drugs

Vitamin deficiency ($B_{12}$, thiamine)

Hypothyroidism

Pick's disease

Neurosyphilis

Paraneoplastic encephalitis

**as an initial evaluation of all patients.** Evaluation should be tailored to the differential diagnosis suggested by the history and exam. **PEARL: Most dementias are not reversible but are improved by identifying treatable causes and by correcting con-**

**current problems.** Such problems may include urinary tract infections, electrolyte disturbances, or adverse drug effects. Clinical imaging studies and pathologic findings (Table 8–2) are the mainstays of classification.

# ALZHEIMER'S DISEASE

Alzheimer's disease is the most common cause of dementia. Prominent features are impairment of new memory, learning, language, and visuospatial function. Apraxias and agnosias are common. Some patients have prominent psychiatric features including paranoia, delusions, depression, and agitation. Patients often retain socially appropriate behavior until the later stages, when insight is lost. Seizures occur in 8%. Focal motor or sensory deficits are uncommon. Gait is preserved until late in the course.

Atrophy is prominent in frontal, temporal, and parietal lobes. Microscopic findings include neuronal loss, neurofibrillary tangles within neurons, and senile plaques in the neuropil. Senile plaques consist of a central core of amyloid surrounded by degenerating neurites. Neurofibrillary tangles, in the form of paired helical filaments, are degenerating neuronal microtubules due to abnormal phosphorylation of tau proteins.

The main neurochemical loss is in the nucleus basalis, the major source of cholinergic innervation to the cerebrum. Other neurotransmitters and neuropeptides depleted include norepinephrine, serotonin, and somatostatin. Severity of dementia best correlates neurochemically with the loss of cholinergic function and pathologically with the loss of neuronal dendritic arborization. Relatives of patients with early-onset AD are at in-

### Table 8–2. LABORATORY WORK-UP
### OF DEMENTIA

| Lab Test | Diagnostic Relevance |
| --- | --- |
| Brain CT | Excludes tumor, subdural hematoma, infarction, hemorrhage, hydrocephalus; atrophy not always correlated with severity of dementia |
| MRI | More sensitive to atrophy, white matter and brainstem lesions than CT |
| Complete blood cell count | Systemic infections, malignancy |
| Liver panel | Hepatic encephalopathy, alcoholism, malignancy |
| Toxicology screen | Detects drug effects, occult recreational drug abuse |
| VDRL | Neurosyphilis |
| EEG | Complex-partial (non-convulsive) status epilepticus, metabolic encephalopathies, Creutzfeldt-Jakob |
| Vitamin $B_{12}$, folate | Vitamin deficiency |
| HIV serology | HIV encephalitis, CMV encephalitis, CNS lymphoma, cerebral toxoplasmosis |
| Lumbar puncture | Neurosyphilis, chronic meningitis, normal pressure hydrocephalus |
| Thyroid function tests, thyroid-stimulating hormone | Hypothyroidism |
| Chest x-ray | Malignancy, infection |
| ECG | Cardiac arrhythmia |
| Genetic probes | Huntington's chorea (Huntington's disease) |

CMV = cytomegalovirus; CT = computed tomography; ECG = electrocardiogram; VDRL = Venereal Disease Research Laboratory.

creased risk of dementia, with an autosomal dominant pedigree in some kindreds. Persons with Down's syndrome (trisomy 21) surviving to the third decade have the neuropathologic changes of AD. An abnormal processing of beta-amyloid, whose gene is located on chromosome 21, is suspected of playing a pathologic role in AD. Other loci for early-onset disease include genes for presenilin-1 and presenilin-2 and a locus on chromosome 12. Apolipoproteins are involved in the metabolism of beta-amyloid; the allele ε4 on chromosome 19 conveys an increased risk of sporadic and familial late-onset AD. Apolipoprotein typing lacks sufficient sensitivity and specificity for diagnosis but may assist in corroborating a clinical diagnosis.

Treatment of AD with cholinergic enhancers is often disappointing. Tetrahydroaminoacridine (Cognex) and donepezil (Aricept) are cholinesterase inhibitors that modestly improve attention, memory, and activities of daily living in those patients who are not yet severely impaired. Cognex is associated with frequent signs of gastrointestinal discomfort and requires frequent laboratory monitoring for chemical hepatitis. Although they do not arrest progression, their use may forestall nursing home placement and "set the clock back" on the neurologic deterioration by about 6 months.

Behavioral symptoms are frequent in AD and merit discussion and treatment. *Agitation* and *psychosis* may respond to risperidone and buspirone. *Anxiety* can be managed with short-acting benzodiazepines (lorazepam), chloral hydrate, buspirone, or trazodone. *Depression* is frequent in the early stages of AD and can be managed with serotonin-specific reuptake inhibitors. Sleep disturbances may respond to physical activity at daycare centers, chloral hydrate, zolpidem, or melatonin.

# MULTI-INFARCT DEMENTIA

*Multi-infarct dementia* ([MID] vascular dementia) accounts for about 15% of cases and is diagnosed with the presence of vascular risk factors (hypertension, diabetes, coronary artery disease) and neuroimaging studies showing focal defects in vascular territories or extensive periventricular white matter loss **(leukoaraiosis).** There is often evidence of vascular insults in other organs, with a history of kidney disease, myocardial infarction, and intermittent claudication. The hallmark of MID is an episodic, stepwise evolution of dementia. However, patients with Binswanger's disease (subacute arteriosclerotic encephalopathy) may exhibit an insidiously progressive decline resembling AD. About 5% of patients have both AD *and* MID.

The exam reveals focal neurologic deficits such as hemiparesis, dysphasia, visual field loss, ataxia, or a gait disturbance. Emotional lability with pseudobulbar palsy (brisk jaw-jerk, hyperactive gag reflex, and spastic dysarthria) may be prominent.

Treatment is aimed at controlling risk factors for vascular disease (hypertension, diabetes, hyperlipidemia) and preventing new cerebrovascular events with antiplatelet agents, anticoagulants, or endarterectomy.

# DIFFUSE LEWY-BODY DEMENTIA

In European series, dementia due to diffuse Lewy-body disease is the second most common cause. There is considerable overlap with Parkinson's disease complicated by dementia. Clinical hallmarks include fluctuating levels of arousal and attention, hallucinations (often visual), extrapyramidal signs (rigidity, bradykinesia), and heightened sensitivity to the extrapyramidal adverse effects of antipsychotic agents.

## OTHER DEMENTIAS

Dementia may be a prominent feature of *Parkinson's disease*, particularly if it occurs in late life. Dementia correlates with the degree of bradykinesia, and patients are unusually sensitive to the behavioral toxicity of antiparkinsonian drugs such as levodopa, bromocriptine, and pergolide.

Dementia may occur in *multiple sclerosis*, especially if white matter in both frontal lobes is involved. In multiple sclerosis, the lesion burden, as shown on magnetic resonance imaging (MRI), correlates more with cognitive decline than with physical decline.

Elderly patients are extremely sensitive to cognitive disturbances caused by many *medicines*, such as antidepressants, tranquilizers, analgesics, and beta-blockers. A thorough medication review and observation while the patient is drug-free is often rewarding.

Frontal and temporal lobe *tumors* such as meningiomas or low-grade gliomas may grow large in clinically silent areas (anterior frontal regions, anterior temporal poles, interhemispheric fissure, and intraventricular regions) and manifest in an advanced state when they cause seizures or raised intracranial pressure. Older patients may develop *subdural hematomas* from ruptured cortical bridging veins, even without a history of significant head injury. Chronic *alcoholism* may cause dementia through several mechanisms: repeated head trauma with contusion to the frontal and temporal poles, thiamine deficiency resulting in

Wernicke-Korsakoff syndrome, cerebral atrophy, and hepatic insufficiency.

*Normal pressure hydrocephalus (NPH)* comprises the clinical triad of gait disturbance ("magnetic gait"), urinary incontinence, and dementia. Diagnosis is supported by the history of an initial gait disturbance and a past history of a central nervous system (CNS) insult (e.g., prior meningitis or subarachnoid or intracerebral hemorrhage that could obstruct drainage through the arachnoid granulations) and improved gait after cerebrospinal fluid (CSF) drainage. When dementia appears in addition to NPH, response to shunt procedures is poor.

Dementia is often an early feature of *Huntington's chorea (Huntington's disease),* and often presents as a psychiatric disturbance. The family history usually reveals that other family members have had the disease. Genetic testing for persons at risk is available.

Most patients with *human immunodeficiency virus (HIV) disease* have CNS involvement at autopsy, and the disorders that can cause the dementia of HIV are legion. Most commonly, HIV causes encephalitis because of CNS infiltration by macrophages harboring the virus. A target cell of CNS involvement by HIV has not been identified. Other common causes include toxoplasmosis, cryptococcal meningitis, cytomegaloviral encephalitis, tuberculous meningitis, and CNS lymphoma. In the absence of HIV infection, *neurosyphilis* is an exceedingly rare cause of dementia. The neurosyphilis of HIV usually is characterized by meningovascular involvement and requires prolonged penicillin therapy.

*Thiamine ($B_1$) deficiency* is mostly seen in alcoholics, some hospitalized patients on chemotherapy and inadequate diets, and those who are starved. Acutely, thiamine deficiency presents as Wernicke's encephalopathy, manifest by the triad of ophthalmoparesis, ataxia, and confusion. Immediate repletion with intravenous thiamine may dramatically reverse the neural deficits. Untreated and unrecognized Wernicke's disease is associated with hemorrhage in the brainstem, and may be fatal. Chronic thiamine deficiency causes Korsakoff's psychosis, characterized by severe short-term memory impairment and confabulation. The short-term memory deficit correlates best with neuronal loss in the dorsomedial thalamus and mamillary bodies.

*Vitamin $B_{12}$ deficiency* may cause severe depression, emotional lability, and attentional impairment, but rarely causes dementia. It is often associated with a large-fiber peripheral neuropathy, posterior column dysfunction ("pseudotabes"), and a megaloblastic anemia (although neural deficits may occur without anemia). Lifelong repletion with $B_{12}$ is indicated.

Mild *impairment of thyroid function* may cause depression. Dementia due to hypothyroidism is accompanied by systemic stigmata of thyroid disease (myxedema, prolonged deep tendon reflex relaxation times, hypothermia, bradycardia). Thyroxine replacement should be gradual, to avoid worsening coronary artery disease or precipitating congestive heart failure.

*Creutzfeldt-Jakob disease (CJD)*, a rare form of dementia, occurs with a uniform worldwide incidence of one per million. It causes a rapidly progressive dementia often associated with myoclonic jerks and periodic epileptiform discharges on electroencephalography (EEG). The etiologic agent is a **prion,** a protein constituent of cell membranes that is altered and catalyzes self-replication. Prion proteins are infectious; inoculating a primate brain with brain tissue from affected patients transmits the disease. Corneal transplants, pituitary extracts, and contaminated neurosurgical equipment have transmitted the disease. *Bovine spongiform encephalopathy* is a CJD variant strain from cattle that is believed to have infected some persons in the United Kingdom.

## PSEUDODEMENTIA

**Pseudodementia** refers to patients with depression associated with reversible intellectual impairment. However, many patients with organic dementias have clinically significant depression, complicating the diagnostic picture. **PEARL: Patients with pseudodementia should have a normal EEG. They also show considerable fluctuation of performance on neuropsychologic testing.** Resolution of cognitive function commensurate with an improved mood supports the diagnosis.

## SYMPTOM MANAGEMENT

Although primary treatment of dementia is dictated by the underlying disorder, many patients also require management of symptoms such as depression or agitation, as already discussed in the section on AD.

The families of demented patients undergo considerable psychological and physical stress. They should be referred to support groups and counseled about options for home care and institutional care. **PEARL: Respite hospitalization for the patient permits family members to recover from the stress of caregiving and may allow the patient to remain in the home setting longer.** Families should seek legal advice about advance directives and wills. Caregivers need to engage in frank discussions about the issues of sedation, feeding, physical restraint, and cardiopulmonary resuscitation.

# 9
## CHAPTER

# *Seizures*

## DEFINITIONS

A **seizure** is a behavioral change resulting from a sudden, excessive, hypersynchronous discharge of cerebral neurons. The behavioral changes are usually stereotyped and may include motor, sensory, autonomic, or mental phenomena as well as changes in level of consciousness. A seizure is a symptom—*not a specific disease*—and can result from various cerebral insults or genetic factors; in many cases, no cause is identified. **Epilepsy** (*seizure disorder*) is diagnosed when a person has two or more seizures without a clear precipitant such as alcohol withdrawal or cocaine use.

## SETTINGS AND MEDICAL PRESENTATION

Seizures most often occur outside the medical setting—at home, school, or work. Most seizures last less than 2 minutes and do not cause convulsive jerking or tonic (rigid) movements. Such brief and nonconvulsive seizures usually are seen in the outpatient setting. Mild convulsions may be mistaken for syncope, although the reverse is more common. When convulsions occur only during sleep and there are no witnesses, a bitten tongue or lip, muscle soreness, or headache on awakening may be the only clues. In some cases, a history of transient unresponsiveness or confusion is obtained incidentally. In contrast, new-onset convulsive tonic-clonic (grand mal) seizures are most often observed in the emergency room.

## DIAGNOSIS

### Patient History

Seizures are diagnosed primarily by the history; descriptions given both by the patient and by observers are valuable. First, try to determine whether the patient had an epileptic seizure or another type of spell. *Seizures* are **paroxysmal** (sudden onset and offset) episodes of behavioral change. Other paroxysmal disorders confused with epilepsy include syncope and conversion disorder (psychogenic seizures; see Chapter 13).

Ask about factors that may have provoked paroxysmal events:
- Sleep deprivation, unusual stress, or recent illness
- Medications or drugs
- Activities just before attack (e.g., rising from a lying position)
- Flickering lights or other stimuli

Ask about characteristics of the attack:
- *Onset:* paroxysmal or gradual.
- *Time at onset:* relation to sleep, waking.
- *Symptoms at onset:* warning, palpitations, nausea, and so forth.

- Abnormal movements (e.g., eyes, mouth, head, arms, or legs).
- Focal features (e.g., unilateral tingling, head deviation).
- *Impairment of consciousness:* Was the ability to talk, respond appropriately, and recall events during the episode impaired?
- Automatisms (e.g., lip smacking, fumbling hand movements).
- Cry or shriek at onset of attack.
- Bowel or bladder incontinence; biting tongue, cheek, or lip.

Ask what occurred after the attack:

- Confusion, lethargy, or need to sleep; duration of postattack symptoms (brief after syncope)
- Headache, muscle soreness, or physical injury
- Focal weakness (Todd's paralysis); sensory or speech impairment

The medical history may reveal a previous brain insult or recent illness that causes seizures, and a general exam may identify disorders associated with seizures (e.g., metabolic and infectious disorders, alcohol withdrawal, neurocutaneous lesions such as adenoma sebaceum in tuberous sclerosis). Orthostatic blood pressure and heart rate changes, heart rhythm, and auscultation of the heart and neck can reveal cardiovascular disorders. The neurologic exam identifies lateralizing or localizing findings.

## Lab Studies

Electroencephalography (EEG), the most specific diagnostic test for epilepsy, measures brain electrical activity. Abnormal patterns may be specific (epileptiform activity) or nonspecific (slowing of the background rhythms from drugs, trauma, stroke, etc.). Abnormalities may be diffuse (generalized spike-and-wave epileptiform discharges or slowing from a sedative overdose) or focal (a spike or slowing restricted to the right temporal area).

Ambulatory EEG uses a portable cassette recorder to study patients for prolonged periods. Video-EEG monitoring allows simultaneous recording of the EEG and the patient's behavior on a split screen. The video-EEG helps to assess patients with spells of uncertain origin (e.g., psychogenic seizures) and helps to localize seizure foci for possible epilepsy surgery.

**PEARL: A normal EEG pattern does not exclude epilepsy.** Because the EEG samples a brief period and only the more superficial cerebral cortex, it rarely records a seizure. **Epileptiform activity** (interictal sharp waves or spikes) or focal slow waves on the EEG support, but do not establish, a diagnosis of epilepsy. The patient's history is the most important diagnostic tool.

A magnetic resonance imaging (MRI) scan should be obtained in all patients with new-onset focal seizures (except for benign rolandic epilepsy of childhood) or tonic-clonic seizures. Lumbar puncture should be performed for patients with possible cerebrospinal fluid (CSF) infection, if there are no contraindications (see Chapter 2).

## CLASSIFICATION

The two major seizure types are *partial* and *generalized* (Table 9–1). Differentiation is critical for diagnosis and treatment. **Partial** (focal) **seizures** begin in one or more restricted cortical areas and mandate a search to exclude a structural brain lesion such as a scar (gliosis) or tumor. Partial

## Table 9–1. CLASSIFICATION OF EPILEPTIC SEIZURES

Partial seizure (focal or local onset)

   Simple partial seizure (consciousness is preserved)

      Motor (focal motor may spread [jacksonian]; versive [eye/head deviation])

      Somatosensory or special sensory (nonstructured hallucinations or illusions in the tactile, visual, auditory, olfactory, gustatory, or vestibular modalities)

      Autonomic (visceral sensations, pallor/flushing, sweating, piloerection, pupillary dilatation)

      Psychic (aphasia, déjà vu, dreamy states, distortion of time, affective changes [fear], illusions, or structured sensory hallucinations)

   Complex partial seizure (consciousness is impaired)

      Arrest of ongoing behavior, stare

      Automatisms common (rubbing hands, lip smacking)

   Simple or complex partial seizure may progress to secondary generalized tonic-clonic seizure

Generalized seizure (bilateral, symmetrical onset)

   Absence seizure

      Typical

      Atypical

   Myoclonic seizure

   Clonic seizure

   Tonic seizure

   Atonic seizure

   Tonic-clonic seizure

seizures are suggested by the clinical history (e.g., an aura of fear or déjà vu), observation (e.g., right arm clonic movements), neuroimaging (e.g., a vascular lesion on MRI), or EEG with focal epileptiform activity.

**Generalized seizures** begin simultaneously in both hemispheres. There are no warnings suggesting local onset, but nonspecific symptoms such as lightheadedness can occur. *Tonic-clonic* (grand mal) *seizures* may be partial or generalized in origin.

## Partial Seizures

**Simple partial seizures** (auras) are usually brief (5 to 180 seconds), include a diverse spectrum of symptoms, affect all ages, and are not associated with impaired consciousness (i.e., patients can respond and remember).

**Complex partial seizures** impair consciousness. The seizure is brief (20 to 180 seconds), but a postictal state with confusion and lethargy often lasts minutes or longer. Most complex partial seizures include automatisms such as lip smacking, chewing, hand rubbing or fumbling.

**Secondary generalized tonic-clonic seizures** resemble generalized tonic-clonic seizures (discussed in the next section), but they begin *focally.*

## Generalized Seizures

**Absence** (petit mal) **seizures** are brief episodes (2 to 20 seconds) of unresponsiveness without aura or postictal symptoms. They usually begin between ages 4 and 14 years. The blank stare may be accompanied by eyeblinks or simple automatisms (e.g., brief lip smacking). The EEG signature of absence seizures is the 3- to 4-Hz spike-and-wave discharge, which is often seen **interictally** (between seizures).

**Atypical absence seizures,** which usually begin in early childhood, are brief periods (5 to 30 seconds) of staring with variable impairment of consciousness. Patients often have atonic and myoclonic seizures as well as mental retardation. The EEG usually shows background slowing and generalized slow (less than 3 Hz) spike-and-slow-wave discharges.

**Myoclonus** is a heterogeneous group of movements characterized by brief, shock-like contractions (jerks) of a muscle or group of muscles. Isolated jerks on falling asleep are normal. Nonepileptic forms result from brainstem lesions (palatal myoclonus), spinal cord lesions (segmental myoclonus), or toxic-metabolic disorders. If myoclonic jerks are bilateral and symmetrical or precede tonic-clonic seizures, they are usually epileptic—that is, *myoclonic seizures* (see juvenile myoclonic epilepsy, discussed in the next section).

**Atonic seizures** produce a sudden loss of postural tone that can cause falls and trauma. These are often refractory to medical therapy.

**Generalized tonic-clonic seizures** (grand mal; convulsions) begin with a brief tonic phase (2 to 10 seconds) with loss of consciousness, extensor rigidity, falling, and often a cry, followed by the clonic phase, with bilateral jerking usually lasting 30 to 180 seconds. There may be cyanosis, hypersalivation, tongue biting, and urinary (less often, fecal) incontinence. Postictally, patients are tired and confused.

## Epilepsy Syndromes

**Epilepsy syndromes** are defined by a cluster of features (seizure types, genetic factors, age of onset, EEG findings). Classifying an epileptic syndrome often provides prognostic and therapeutic information. Two common examples are juvenile myoclonic epilepsy and temporal lobe epilepsy.

**Juvenile myoclonic epilepsy** is defined by myoclonic seizures with or without tonic-clonic or absence seizures. Seizures usually begin between ages 8 and 18 years and most often occur in the early morning, shortly after awaking. Generalized spike-and-slow-wave discharges are commonly seen. Seizures are usually well controlled with valproate. Carbamazepine and phenytoin can worsen myoclonic and absence seizures.

**Temporal lobe epilepsy** is a partial epilepsy syndrome in which simple (autonomic, visceral, and psychic) and complex partial seizures predominate. Many patients have a history of febrile seizures. MRI often reveals mesial temporal sclerosis (cell loss in the hippocampus). Patients refractory to medications often benefit from surgery.

## TREATMENT

Tables 9–2 and 9–3 summarize the medications used for epilepsy. Control is the seizure-free state or the occasional occurrence of seizures that do not interfere with the patient's life. **PEARL: The benefits of seizure control must be balanced against the side effects of antiepileptic drugs (AEDs): Seizures are infrequent, but AED treatment is continuous.**

### Initiating Therapy

Antiepileptic drug therapy should begin with a single drug. Gradually increase dosage until control is achieved or side effects are bothersome. The efficacy of a drug and meaningful serum level can only be assessed in steady state.

### Increasing the Dose

Once low therapeutic levels are reached, the dose should be increased slowly if seizures persist. Because of phenytoin's kinetics, a small dose in-

### Table 9–2. TREATMENT OF SEIZURE
### BY TYPE*

Partial seizure (simple, complex, and secondary generalized)

*Drugs of choice:* carbamazepine, phenytoin

*Alternative choices:* gabapentin, lamotrigine, oxcar-
bazepine, phenobarbital, primidone, tiagabine,
topiramate, valproate

Absence seizure (without tonic-clonic seizure)

*Drug of choice:* ethosuximide

*Alternative choices:* valproate (acetazolamide, clonazepam,
lamotrigine)

Absence seizure (with tonic-clonic seizure)

*Drug of choice:* valproate

*Alternative choices:* ethosuximide, lamotrigine
(acetazolamide, clonazepam)

Generalized tonic-clonic seizure

*Drug of choice:* valproate

*Alternative choices:* carbamazepine, lamotrigine, phenytoin,
topiramate (phenobarbital, primidone)

*Drugs are listed in alphabetical order. Those in parentheses
are third-line drugs.

crease may cause a large increase in serum levels.
For example, a patient taking 300 mg/day of
phenytoin may have a blood level of 14 µg/mL; if
the dosage is increased to 400 mg/day, the blood
level could increase to a toxic 30 µg/mL. In this
case, an increase of only 25 to 50 mg/day would be
better.

## Checking Antiepileptic Drug Levels

**PEARL: Treat the patient, not the blood level.**  Levels monitor compliance and guide therapy; they
are not mandates to change the dose. If a patient
is "subtherapeutic" but seizure-free, there is usually no reason to increase the dose. If the patient's

## Table 9–3. COMMON DRUGS FOR TREATMENT OF EPILEPSY

| Drug (Trade Name) | Usual Adult Daily Dose (mg) | Dosing Interval | Therapeutic Range (Serum) (µg/mL) | Plasma Half-Life (h) | Toxicity |
|---|---|---|---|---|---|
| Acetazolamide (Diamox) | 375–1000 | bid–tid | — | 12 | Paresthesia, diuresis, renal stones |
| Carbamazepine (Tegretol; sustained-release Tegretol XR) | 600–1600 | bid–qid | 6–12 | 6–12 (with chronic use; 14 h with extended release) | Sedation, rash, GI discomfort, hypercholesterolemia, hepatic and marrow toxicity |
| Clonazepam (Klonopin) | 0.5–3 | qd–tid | — | 35 | Drowsiness, unsteadiness, behavioral changes |
| Ethosuximide (Zarontin) | 750–2250 | bid–tid | 40–100 | 24–48 (approx. 30 in children, 40 in adults) | GI discomfort, sedation, ataxia, hepatic and marrow toxicity |
| Gabapentin (Neurontin) | 1800–3600 | tid | >2 | 6–8 | Tiredness, dizziness, unsteadiness, weight gain |
| Lamotrigine (Lamictal) | 150–6000 | bid–tid | 1–20 | 30 | Rash, nausea, insomnia, dizziness, unsteadiness, diplopia |
| Oxcarbazepine (Trileptal) | 600–2400 | bid | ? | 6–10 (active metabolite) | |

**Table 9–3. COMMON DRUGS FOR TREATMENT OF EPILEPSY**

| Drug (Trade Name) | Usual Adult Daily Dose (mg) | Dosing Interval | Therapeutic Range (Serum μg/mL) | Plasma Half-Life (h) | Toxicity |
|---|---|---|---|---|---|
| Phenobarbital (Luminal) | 90–250 | qd (bedtime) | 15–40 | 90–100 | Sedation, cognitive slowing, irritability, depression, impotence, rash |
| Phenytoin (Dilantin) | 250–450 | qd–tid | 10–20 | 14–26 | Rash, unsteadiness, hirsutism, sedation, gingival hyperplasia |
| Primidone (Mysoline); metabolized to phenobarbital | 750–1500 | bid–qid | 5–15 (phenobarbital 5–35) | 16–18 (phenobarbital 90–110) | (Same as phenobarbital) |
| Tiagabine (Gabatril) | 32–56 | bid–qid | — | 4–8 | Dizziness, tiredness, nausea, irritability, tremor |
| Topiramate (Topamax) | 100–500 | bid | ? | 18–24 | Drowsiness, dizziness, anxiety, mental slowing, |
| Valproate (Depakene; delayed-release Depakote) | 750–3500 | bid–qid | 25–125 | 12–18 (slow release, 24) | Nausea, vomiting, tremor, hair loss, weight gain, hepatic toxocity, thrombocytopenia, pancreatitis, menstrual irregularities |

level is "upper therapeutic" but he or she still has seizures, a dose increase may be indicated if toxicity is minimal. Levels are usually obtained at a trough (shortly before the next dose) to provide greater consistency between measures. The frequency of obtaining AED levels is guided by the clinical picture. For well-controlled patients, once a year is sufficient.

## Changing Antiepileptic Drugs

If the first AED is unsuccessful because of adverse affects, another AED monotherapy should be used. Introduce the new drug slowly while tapering off the first drug (make sure one is always at therapeutic levels). If the second AED trial is unsuccessful, or if the first AED fails to control seizures with therapeutic levels, two-drug therapy should be considered.

## The Single Seizure

Evaluation and treatment of patients with a single seizure are controversial. Patients reporting their first absence or partial seizure often have had previous episodes that are discovered by a thorough history from the patient and observers. Tonic-clonic seizures are rarely missed unless they occur during sleep or are not witnessed.

Treatment decisions are difficult for patients with a single tonic-clonic seizure. The recurrence rate varies from 16% to 61%, and is higher with a history of brain injury or abnormality, partial onset, abnormal findings on neurologic exam, or epileptiform activity on EEG. Seizures most often recur within the first year. If someone has had two seizures, the risk is 85% that he or she will have a third.

Therapy is usually deferred after a single seizure if no risk factors are present. (Risk of recurrence is approximately 20%.) Treatment decisions are complex and influenced by the number of risk factors, timing of the seizure during the sleep-wake cycle (a recurrence is more likely to occur in the same state), the patient's need to drive or operate dangerous equipment, and so forth.

## Danger Signs for a Patient with Epilepsy

Patients should be reassessed (and, in some cases, reimaged with MRI) if they develop:
- New headaches (e.g., positional, increased with Valsalva's maneuver, unrelated to seizures)
- Increased seizure frequency unexplained by poor compliance, change in drug levels, pregnancy, and so forth
- A new type of seizure or postictal deficit
- New focal neurologic deficits or focal EEG slowing

## Follow-up of the Chronic Seizure Patient

On routine visits, patients should be questioned and examined to determine:
- Seizure frequency (noted in a seizure diary, recording possible precipitating factors such as time of day, menstrual cycle, etc.)
- Medication toxicity
- Cognitive function
- Mood (depression is common)
- Quality of life (how they believe they are doing)

## The Refractory Patient

Patients treated with two AEDs who have documented therapeutic trough AED levels and persistent seizures should be considered for referral to an epilepsy center. Try to identify possible precipitating factors (e.g., alcohol, sleep deprivation, noncompliance) or atypical features (duration more than 5 minutes, preserved consciousness despite bilateral tonic or clonic activity) suggesting psychogenic seizures. Surgical therapy can help many patients with refractory epilepsy.

## Remission and Antiepileptic Drug Withdrawal

After epilepsy is diagnosed and treated, two-thirds of patients become seizure-free for 5 years. The longer is the time interval, the greater the chance of remission. Factors predicting a higher remission rate include normal findings on exam, MRI, and EEG; primary generalized tonic-clonic seizures; and younger age when epilepsy is diagnosed. Consider AED withdrawal after a 2-year seizure-free interval. AEDs should be gradually tapered over months (more than 1 to 3 months for barbiturates, depending on the dose).

# 10

CHAPTER

# *Movement and Gait Disorders*

Movement and gait disorders are heterogenous and result from dysfunction at any anatomic level (from cortex to neuromuscular junction) or system level (pyramidal to sensory). **PEARL: Before diagnosing a syndrome involving a movement disorder, carefully define the symptom.** Movement disorders can result from loss of normal function, such as weakness or impaired coordination, or from adventitious (extra) movements, such as tremor, dyskinesia, or chorea. After the patient or witness describes the symptom, ask him or her to imitate it, if possible. Then, observe the patient. Record the observed and described clinical features (e.g., hand is held in sustained, partial flexion of an unnatural posture, which is uncomfortable but not painful, etc.). Determine what factors exacerbate or improve the symptom.

**PEARL: After defining the symptom, consider different lesion sites that could cause the symptom.** Search for associated motor, sensory, or other features that help to define the anatomy.

# COMMON SYMPTOMS OF MOVEMENT DISORDERS

## Weakness

When weakness is observed in the outpatient setting, the time course, distribution of involved muscles, and associated neurologic findings help to determine the anatomic site and etiology. Causes of sudden-onset or rapidly progressing weakness are reviewed in Chapter 15. **PEARL: Decreased dexterity out of proportion to weakness distinguishes upper motor neuron disorders (and cerebellar and extrapyramidal causes) from lower motor neuron disorders.** In the clinic, other important causes of weakness are:

- Nerve entrapment ("pinched" nerve or nerve root; e.g., sciatica with foot weakness, carpal tunnel syndrome [see Chapter 7])
- Polyneuropathy (e.g., diabetes [see Chapter 7])
- Multiple sclerosis (MS [see Chapter 11])
- Myasthenia gravis
- Brain or spinal cord tumor (see Chapter 21)

Evaluation depends on the suspected anatomy and cause. (See Chapter 15.)

## Spasticity

Lesions of the frontal lobe motor cortex or corticospinal tract cause weakness and spasticity (decreased dexterity, increased tone and deep tendon reflexes, clonus, Babinski's sign, flexor spasms). Common causes include stroke, tumor, MS, and trauma. Spasticity usually develops weeks after an acute neurologic event (e.g., stroke) or with chronic progressive disorders (e.g., MS, tumor).

In the clinic, most patients with spasticity have a history of prior neurologic disease, but it may be an important clue to an undiagnosed lesion (e.g., a spinal cord tumor).

### *Treatment*

Spasticity can respond to drugs, especially with spinal cord lesions and when associated with flexor spasms. Baclofen, tinazidine, and benzodiazepines are considered first-line agents in treating spasticity due to spinal cord disease, MS, and cerebral palsy. *Baclofen* (Lioresal; gamma-aminobutyric acid [$GABA_B$] receptor agonist) is started at 5 mg bid and increased to 20 to 80 mg/day; weakness and sedation limit dose. *Tinazidine* (Zanaflex, alpha$_2$-agonist) is started at 2 mg tid and increased to 36 mg/day; sedation and dry mouth are common side effects. *Diazepam* (Valium; $GABA_A$ receptor agonist) is a commonly used benzodiazepine.

*Dantrolene* (Dantrium) interferes with excitation-contraction of muscle fiber by inhibiting calcium release. Because it causes weakness, it is most useful for bedridden or wheelchair-bound patients.

Intrathecal baclofen can be used when oral drugs fail.

## Parkinsonism

Parkinsonism presents with various combinations of:

- **Bradykinesia** (slowness and impaired initiation of movement).
- Increased tone ("lead-pipe" rigidity). Muscle tension is fairly consistent throughout the range of movement; there is resistance to movement in all directions. "Cogwheel rigidity" results from superimposed tremor.

- A resting tremor that is often coarse.
- Expressionless (masked) facies, diminished blinking.
- Shuffling, slow gait. The trunk is often flexed, arm swing is decreased, and postural balance is impaired. Patients may also have a **festinating gait** (the tendency to accelerate their pace as they appear to chase their center of gravity).
- Impaired postural reflexes with frequent falls.
- Depression and mild cognitive impairment.

### *Causes*

Parkinsonism is often induced by drugs (e.g., dopamine-receptor blockers such as haloperidol and metoclopramide). **PEARL: Drug-induced parkinsonism cannot be distinguished clinically from Parkinson's disease. These patients must be observed for improvement when not taking the drug.** A common degenerative disorder, **Parkinson's disease** features progressive loss of substantia nigra and other pigmented brainstem nuclei. Less common degenerative disorders with similar symptoms include *progressive supranuclear palsy,* which is associated with defective conjugate gaze (vertical gaze more impaired than horizontal) and mild dementia; *Shy-Drager syndrome,* which is associated with autonomic impairment (orthostatic hypotension); and *striatonigral degeneration,* which responds poorly to dopaminergic therapy.

### *Treatment*

*Levodopa* (a precursor of dopamine), the first-line treatment of Parkinson's disease, is given with a peripheral dopa decarboxylase inhibitor (*carbidopa*) to reduce non–central nervous system (CNS) side effects such as hypotension, nausea, and arrhythmias. Carbidopa-levodopa in combination (Sinemet) is available as 10 mg carbidopa and 100 mg levodopa (10/100), 25/100, and 25/250 tablets. A long-acting form (25/100 or 50/200) is also available. The initial dose is usually 25/100 tid.

Peak-dose adverse effects of levodopa include nausea and vomiting, dyskinesias (usually chorea, discussed later), agitation, confusion, vivid dreaming, hallucinations, and psychosis. As an end-of-dose wearing-off effect, parkinsonian symptoms worsen shortly before the next dose is due. That effect can be improved by using a controlled-release preparation, increasing the frequency of dosing, or decreasing the dose.

Dopamine agonists can reduce the "on-off" phenomenon, which occurs with prolonged levodopa therapy and is characterized by variable periods (20 to 150 minutes) of severe bradykinesia, hypotonia, and fear, which can begin and end abruptly. Dopamine agonists (e.g., *bromocriptine* [Parlodel] and *pergolide*) directly stimulate dopamine receptors, often allowing a reduction of levodopa dosage, and reducing end-of-dose wearing-off effect and peak-dose side effects (e.g., dyskinesias).

*Amantadine* (Symmetrel) releases dopamine stored at nerve endings.

*Selegiline* is a selective monamine oxidase B (MAO-B) inhibitor that can forestall or reduce the need for levodopa therapy. Selegiline may be neuroprotective, preventing the degeneration of nigrostriatal neurons, but this effect is not proved. Dietary restriction of tyramine is not needed.

*Anticholinergics* are usually only helpful for the prominent tremor of early stages of Parkinson's disease. These drugs commonly cause dry mouth, blurred vision, dizziness, and constipation. The anticholinergics include benztropine (Cogentin) and trihexyphenidyl (Artane).

The role of *surgeries* such as fetal transplant and medial pallidotomy is still being defined in selected cases.

## Akathisia

**Akathisia** is a condition of restlessness, inability to sit still (legs and arms may move continuously as if driven by a motor), and anxiety. Akathisia most often develops after chronic treatment with dopamine blockers. Beta-blockers, anticholinergics, and dose reduction or drug discontinuation are helpful.

## Chorea and Athetosis

**Chorea** refers to involuntary movements of the extremities that are rapid, jerky, irregular, and give the appearance of restlessness. The movements often begin and end suddenly. **Athetosis** refers to slow, nearly continuous writhing movements of the distal extremities. In several neurologic disorders, chorea and athetosis are combined and are termed **choreoathetosis.** If chorea is severe and persistent, it becomes difficult to distinguish from athetosis.

Chorea can occur with thyrotoxicosis, pregnancy, lupus, stroke, estrogen drugs, and acute rheumatic fever (Sydenham's chorea). Treat the primary disorder. **Huntington's chorea** (Huntington's disease) is an autosomal dominant inherited degenerative disease that causes personality changes, dementia, chorea, and athetosis. Symptoms usually begin between the ages of 15 and 40. Drugs that deplete dopamine (tetrabenazine, reserpine) or block dopamine receptors (haloperidol, chlorpromazine) may be helpful.

## Tardive Dyskinesia

**Tardive dyskinesia** is a condition of involuntary chorealike movements of the face, sometimes the neck, and a limb after more than 6 months of antipsychotic treatment with dopamine blockers. It is more prevalent in women than in men. Chewing and lip smacking, tongue movements, and facial grimacing are most common. Tardive dyskinesia is aggravated by anticholinergics. The condition is often refractory to treatment and may be permanent. The treatment is gradual reduction of antipsychotic dosage. Tetrabenazine (Nitoman, not available in United States), reserpine (Serpasil), valproate (Depakote), or baclofen (Lioresal) may be used as adjuncts. Tetrabenazine and reserpine may work by reducing dopaminergic activity; valproate and baclofen, by increasing GABAergic activity.

## Dystonia

**Dystonia** is a condition of involuntary, sustained muscle contraction, most often of the trunk, proximal extremities, or eyelids. *Focal dystonia* is most common and involves selected muscle groups:
- *Torticollis:* neck muscles
- *Blepharospasm:* eyelids
- *Meige's syndrome:* eye and facial muscles
- *Writer's cramp:* hand muscles

*Acute* dystonia usually occurs within the first week of therapy with a dopaminergic blocker and is more common in men than in women. Such cases are seen in the outpatient clinic or emergency room or occur on a medical or psychiatric ward. The offending drug should be stopped. *Chronic* dystonia is most often a sporadic illness seen in the outpatient clinic, but it can also result from metabolic or genetic disorders.

Generalized dystonia is treated with anticholinergics, diphenhydramine (for dopamine blockers), benzodiazepines, and antispastic drugs. Local injection of botulinum A toxin (Botox) can effectively treat focal dystonia for weeks to months, and then additional injections can be used.

## Tic Disorders

**Tics** are rapid, coordinated movements that resemble purposeful acts. Although involuntary, there is often a compulsion to perform them, but tics can be briefly suppressed. *Motor tics* vary from simple movements (e.g., rapid head deviation, eye blinks) to complex acts (e.g., banging arms on legs as if drumming). *Vocal tics* vary from simple coughs and throat-clearing grunts to cursing **(coprolalia).**

**Tourette's syndrome** is a chronic motor and vocal tic disorder that usually begins between the ages of 3 and 14. Obsessive-compulsive behaviors and attention deficit hyperactivity disorder are common in patients with Tourette's. Tics and behavioral symptoms are treated with haloperidol (Haldol), pimozide (Orap), risperidone (Risperidal),or tetrabenazine (Nitoman). Clonidine (Catapres) and selective serotonin reuptake inhibitors (e.g., fluoxetine [Prozac], sertraline, paroxetine) can help behavioral symptoms.

## Tremor

A **tremor** is an involuntary, rhythmic, repetitive oscillatory shaking movement of the extremities or head. Its classification relies on clinical features, such as the areas of the body affected, frequency of oscillation (rate in hertz), and amplitude, relying on the setting of maximal tremor.

*Resting tremor* is associated with Parkinson's disease. The sustained postural tremor **(action tremor)** may be observed when patients extend their arms in front of their chest. Action tremor is usually classified as an *essential tremor* (onset before age 65 without a family history) or as a systemic disorder. Tremor seen only with volitional movements **(intention tremor)** is most often associated with cerebellar disorders, but parkinsonian and essential tremor are much more common and can also be present (but not maximal) with movement.

### Action Tremor

*Action tremors* are most often seen as a prominent complaint in outpatients, but they are also common in hospitalized patients. Action tremors most often affect the hand. Their frequency is 7 to 14 Hz, and their amplitude is usually low (i.e., a fine tremor, as opposed to the coarse, higher-amplitude tremor of Parkinson's disease). The tremor is usually symmetrical.

#### Causes

Causes of action tremor include:
- *Physiologic:* This occurs with movements requiring sustained posture and precision and is commonly seen with fatigue and anxiety.
- *Metabolic or endocrine disorders* such as uremia, liver disease, drug withdrawal, hypoglycemia, or thyrotoxicosis.
- *Drugs* such as catecholaminergic agents (amphetamines, beta-agonists), steroids, thyroxine, valproate, theophylline, caffeine, tricyclic antidepressants, antipsychotics, and lithium.
- *Familial* tremor (family history present).
- *Senile* tremor (onset after age 65).
- *Essential* tremor (onset before age 65 without family history).

**Treatment**

Action tremor may be treated with *propranolol* (Inderal or other beta-blockers) at an initial dose of 20 mg tid, or 80 mg of a long-acting preparation, which may be increased to 320 mg/day as needed and tolerated.

*Primidone* (Mysoline, 50 to 500 mg/day) can also be helpful.

## Impaired Coordination (Ataxia)

Impaired coordination **(ataxia)** must be carefully assessed to distinguish common causes such as weakness and sensory loss **(proprioceptive deficit)** from pure coordination defect (usually due to lesions in the cerebellum or its connections).

*Acute onset* of impaired coordination often is seen in the emergency room, but can also be seen in the clinic. Diagnostic possibilities include:
- Stroke
- Inflammatory polyneuropathy (e.g., Guillain-Barré syndrome)
- Trauma
- MS

However, all of these can occur more gradually (subacute course).

Chronic and gradually progressive causes of ataxia include:
- Polyneuropathy
- Tumor
- Metabolic (e.g., alcohol)
- Hereditary and degenerative spinocerebellar disorders (e.g., Friedreich's ataxia, olivopontocerebellar atrophy [OPCA])
- MS

Lesions of the cerebellum and its connections are common causes of isolated ataxia. The midline portions of the cerebellum are involved with gait and trunk movements; the lateral cerebellar hemispheres help to coordinate movements of the distal limbs and speech. Lesions of the cerebellum or of its connections cause:

- *Ataxia:* unsteadiness; tested with tandem gait
- *Intention tremor:* worse with volitional movements such as reaching for an object; tested by finger-to-nose or heel-to-shin tests
- **Dysmetria:** inability to gauge distance, power, or speed of a movement; causes overshoot and undershoot movements
- **Asynergy:** lack of coordination between muscle groups; movements are awkward and disjointed
- **Dysdiadochokinesis:** impaired ability to stop one action and immediately follow it by the opposite action; tested by having patients alternately tap the palm and dorsum of their hand
- *Mild weakness and fatigability*
- *Speech disorders:* slurred, jerky, rapid, or staccato speech; marked changes in volume ("explosive")
- *Hypotonia*
- *Diminished deep tendon reflexes:* when the knee-jerk is elicited, a pendulum-like movement of the leg may result (pendular reflex)

# GAIT

## Normal Gait

**Gait** is a complex, fluid movement integrating multiple neurologic systems. The body is erect, the arms dangle loosely and move synchronously with the opposite leg, the medial malleoli nearly touch as the legs pass, and the heel strikes the ground first.

## History and Exam of Gait Disorders

The history and physical exam attempt to identify the anatomy and causes of gait impairment. Before assuming a neurologic cause of gait impairment, determine whether pain (arthritis, fracture) or other disorders limit gait. **PEARL: Gait disorders may occur as isolated neurologic defects (e.g., midline cerebellar, spinocerebellar, or frontal lesions) but are usually associated with other neurologic symptoms and signs:**

- *Headache* leads to suspicion of an intracranial process such as hydrocephalus or tumor.
- *Double vision and vertigo* lead to suspicion of brainstem, cerebellar, or labyrinthine disorder.
- *Back pain* leads to suspicion of spinal cord compression.
- *Incontinence* leads to suspicion of intracranial or intraspinal disorders, or a peripheral nerve disorder such as diabetes.

Gait disorders may involve multiple factors, especially in the elderly. These include impaired sensation (vestibular, visual, proprioceptive), motor dysfunction (pyramidal, extrapyramidal), rheumatologic and orthopedic problems (joint stiffness and pain in the spine and legs), and orthostatic disturbances.

When taking the patient *history*, determine the nature of the gait problem and the settings most often associated with it (e.g., walking up or down stairs, walking in the dark, running).

The *exam* should screen for dysfunction at anatomic sites associated with gait impairment: muscle, neuromuscular junction, nerve root, spinal cord, cerebellum, basal ganglia, frontal or parietal cortex (see Chapter 1). Observe the patient standing and walking spontaneously. Note whether the gait is stiff or fluid (Table 10–1). Note any discomfort, flexion of the trunk, unsteadiness, de-

**Table 10–1. CLINICAL FEATURES OF GAIT DISORDERS**

| Type of Disorder | Leg Movements | Base | Arm Swing | Tandem Gait | Weakness | Sensory Loss | Reflexes |
|---|---|---|---|---|---|---|---|
| STIFF OR SPASTIC | | | | | | | |
| Parkinson's | Slow, short, hesitating, shuffling | Narrow | Decreased: bilateral or unilateral | Mildly impaired | Absent | Absent | Normal |
| Hemiplegic | Circumduction | Slightly wide | Decreased: unilateral | Impaired | Yes | Variable | Increased |
| Frontal lobe | Slow, short, hesitating, shuffling | Slightly to moderately wide | Decreased: bilateral | Impaired | Absent or mild | Absent | Increased |
| NOT STIFF | | | | | | | |
| Cerebellar | Unsteady | Wide | Normal | Severely impaired | None | Absent | Normal |
| Sensory (proprioceptive) | Awkward, unsteady; foot slaps on ground | Wide | Normal | Impaired, severely with eyes closed | Absent | Yes | Absent |

| | | | | | | |
|---|---|---|---|---|---|---|
| Choreo-athetoid | Extraneous movements, slow, awkward | Narrow or slightly wide | Normal to slightly decreased; jerks | Normal, mildly impaired | Absent; movements are clumsy | None | Normal |
| Steppage | Excessive hip flexion | Normal or slightly wide | Normal | Mildly impaired | Footdrop | Absent | Ankle jerk absent; others often absent |
| Conversion (hysteria; astasia-abasia) | May drag foot or extremely unsteady | Variable | Normal | Usually impaired | Variable | Variable | Normal |

creased arm swing, stiffness or flexion of an arm, posturing (such as the fingers curling up), step length, ease of turning, distance between the feet as they pass each other, and how and where the foot strikes the ground.

Ask the patient to walk a straight line (placing one foot in front of the other) with the heel touching the toe. Note unsteadiness. Ask the patient to stand with feet together, first with the eyes open and then closed. Significantly increased swaying with eyes closed **(Romberg's sign)** suggests a proprioceptive deficit compensated for by vision; unsteadiness with eyes both open and closed suggests a cerebellar disorder. Wild lurching movements without fall or a history of injury suggests *astasia-abasia,* a conversion symptom.

# *11*
## CHAPTER

# *Multiple Sclerosis*

## EPIDEMIOLOGY AND ETIOLOGY

Multiple sclerosis (MS) is the leading cause of acquired chronic neurologic disability in young adults, with usual onset between ages 16 and 40; 5% have onset after 50 years, often with a progressive myelopathy. Women are affected twice as often as men. In the United States, prevalence is about 0.1%, affecting an estimated 350,000 persons. The incidence seems to increase with increasing latitude, perhaps partially because MS is most common in whites of northern European descent. Migration studies suggest that risk is determined by latitude of residence before age 15.

Both environmental and genetic factors play a role in MS. The concordance rate in monozygotic twins is about 30%, versus 6% in dizygotic twins. MS is regarded as an autoimmune disorder triggered in genetically susceptible persons by viral infection. Target antigens include myelin basic protein, proteolipid protein, myelin-associated glycoprotein, and myelin-oligodendrocyte glycoprotein.

# PATHOLOGY

Multiple sclerosis is characterized by inflammatory demyelination of the central nervous system (CNS). Inflammation is perivenular in plaques. Immunoglobulin from plasma cells, detected as oligoclonal banding in the cerebrospinal fluid (CSF), may opsonize myelin for endocytosis by activated macrophages. Recent evidence suggests that axonal loss is another prominent process, occurring early in the disease and in normal-appearing white matter. Accumulating axonal loss, along with progressive gliosis, underlies the development of irreversible neural deficits.

# CLINICAL SYMPTOMS

Common symptoms of MS, in order of frequency, include weakness, visual loss (optic neuritis), sensory loss or paresthesias, brainstem dysfunction, incoordination, ataxia of limbs or trunk, fatigue, bladder disturbances, sexual dysfunction, **Lhermitte's sign** (dorsal paresthesias provoked by neck flexion), neuralgia, and cognitive and emotional disturbances (depression). Clinical signs are referable to disturbance in central myelin and can include optic pallor or atrophy, internuclear opthalmopareses, dysarthria, hyperreflexia and spasticity, pyramidal weakness and paraparesis, cerebellar tremor, vibratory sense loss, clonus, and Babinski signs. Dementia, aphasia, seizures, and extrapyramidal symptoms are rare as initial manifestations.

Multiple sclerosis commonly occurs in **exacerbations** (episodes of worsening, also called **"flares"**), in which new symptoms of CNS dysfunction appear within hours to days. Increased core body temperature (e.g., fever, prolonged exercise) worsens neural function transiently (**"pseudoexacerbations"**). The only confirmed triggers of flare-ups are prior infections (usually viral upper respiratory infections) and the 3 to 9 months postpartum. Apparent clinical stability is misleading: Autopsy studies and repeated neuroimaging demonstrate widespread active lesions, many of which are clinically "silent."

## CLINICAL COURSE

The clinical course of MS is extremely variable. The average patient has up to two exacerbations annually; their frequency tends to decline over time. Most flare-ups recur in areas of prior clinical involvement. Twenty-five percent of patients display a **relapsing-remitting pattern** of relatively stable functioning between discrete exacerbations. Over time, 50% of patients become **secondarily progressive,** gradually accumulating disability after an initially relapsing-remitting pattern. Smaller numbers of patients experience continuous worsening from the start with or without clear-cut exacerbations.

## DIAGNOSTIC CRITERIA AND LABORATORY TESTING

The fundamental criterion for diagnosis is separation of lesions in time and in space:
- Symptoms should be consistent with CNS white matter dysfunction.
- Attacks should be separated by at least 1 month.

- Multiple lesions should occur in separate parts of the CNS.
- There should be objective deficits on examination.
- Investigation excludes other medical or neurologic disorders (see "Differential Diagnoses and Prognoses").

MS is sometimes classified as *clinically definite, lab supported, probable, and possible* depending on the history of attacks, signs on exam, and lab abnormalities (magnetic resonance imaging [MRI], oligoclonal banding) supporting the diagnosis. **PEARL: In the absence of a pathognomic biomarker, MS remains a *clinical* diagnosis. An abnormal MRI, without convincing clinical symptoms or signs, cannot be used to make the diagnosis. Conversely, a normal MRI of the brain and spinal cord, with a compatible history or exam, does *not* exclude the diagnosis.**

Cerebrospinal fluid may reveal a mild lymphocytic pleocytosis. *Protein* may be slightly elevated, but should be less than 1 g/L; *glucose* levels are normal. CSF Venereal Disease Research Laboratory (VDRL) testing should be performed. *Oligoclonal banding* by immunoelectrophoresis is positive in up to 90% of persons with definite MS. CSF immunoglobulin G levels and synthesis, myelin basic protein, and kappa light chains are ancillary, corroborative assays.

*Evoked potentials* identify clinically silent white matter lesions and document dissemination in space (i.e., whether different parts of the CNS are affected). Patients may have significant defects along visual, somatosensory, and brainstem pathways without clinical symptoms or signs. Visual evoked potentials are the most helpful.

*Magnetic resonance imaging* is the most sensitive study for diagnosing MS, indicating lesions in about 80% of patients. MRI of the brain and spinal cord provides evidence of clinically silent lesions and excludes other diagnoses or complicating conditions (e.g., cervical spondylosis). MRI signals are mainly confined to the white matter, with a predilection for the periventricular regions. Corpus callosum lesions, best seen on sagittal views, are virtually pathognomonic of MS. Gadolinium enhancement identifies active lesions. MRI lesion morphology overlaps changes seen with cerebrovascular disease and normal aging. **PEARL: T2-weighted lesions are nonspecific and can be related to edema, inflammation, demyelination, gliosis, remyelination, or axonal loss. T1-weighted lesions without gadolinium enhancement ("black holes") are more specifically indicative of axonal loss or gliosis and correlate better with physical disability measures.** Fluid-attenuated-inversion-recovery (FLAIR) images enhance T2 lesion resolution, especially in the spinal cord. The contribution of myelin loss versus axonal loss to brain atrophy in MS is not differentiated by current MRI measures. After a clinically isolated demyelinating episode (optic neuritis, brainstem syndrome, transverse myelitis), an abnormal MRI indicating clinically silent lesions increases the risk of developing clinically definite MS within 5 years by several-fold.

## DIFFERENTIAL DIAGNOSIS AND PROGNOSIS

Other disorders that resemble MS usually can be differentiated based on the history, exam, and specific lab testing. Persons with MS are vulnerable to concurrent conditions, of course, so when the clinical course is atypical, appropriate neuroimaging studies and other tests are indicated. Table 11–1 lists common entities in the differential diagnosis and their clinical discriminating features.

## Table 11–1. DIFFERENTIAL DIAGNOSES
## OF MULTIPLE SCLEROSIS

| Clinical Entity | Discriminating Features |
| --- | --- |
| Acute disseminated encephalomyelitis | Monophasic course; recent viral infection or vaccination; prior measles infection |
| Spinocerebellar degenerations | Pedigree analysis; insidiously progressive course; symmetric involvement; atrophy without demyelination or gadolinium enhancement on MRI; normal CSF |
| HIV encephalopathy | HIV antibody positive; subcortical dementia; diffuse subcortical gray- and white-matter involvement on MRI |
| Tropical spastic paraparesis | Caribbean/Asian ethnicity; HTLV-I serology |
| Progressive multifocal leukoencephalopathy | CT and MRI lesions are non-enhancing; no oligoclonal banding; prominent dementia and aphasia; underlying immunosuppression always present (e.g., HIV, post-transplantation chemotherapy) |
| Compressive myelopathies (cervical spondylosis, Arnold-Chiari malformation) | Revealed by MRI of spinal cord and craniocervical junction; lower motor neuron signs in upper limbs; lower cranial nerve palsies |
| Intracranial tumors (gliomas, lymphomas) | Course gradually increasing in severity; recurrent seizures; normal evoked potentials or lumbar puncture |
| Systemic lupus, other collagen-vascular diseases (Sjögren's syndrome, Behçet's disease) | Organ involvement outside CNS; abnormal serology (e.g., antinuclear antibodies, complement levels) |
| Neurosarcoidosis | Rare without extra-CNS clinical involvement; peripheral facial palsy common; reduced glucose in CSF; elevated angiotensin levels in CSF and serum |

| | |
|---|---|
| Cerebral autosomal dominant arteriopathy with subcortical infarcts and leukoencephalopathy | Mendelian pedigree; classic lacunar or brainstem stroke syndromes; spinal cord lesions extremely rare |
| Craniocervical-junction anomalies | Revealed by MRI of craniocervical junction; lower cranial nerve palsies |
| Neurosyphilis | Serum and CSF VDRL; reflex loss in tabes |
| Central pontine myelinolysis | Dysarthria, dysphagia, ophthalmoparesis, quadriparesis; rapidly corrected hyponatremia |
| Subacute combined degeneration | Low serum vitamin $B_{12}$ levels; risk factors for serum $B_{12}$ malabsorption |
| Neuroborreliosis (Lyme disease) | History of erythema chronicum migrans, facial palsy, radiculopathy, arthropathy; positive serum and CSF Lyme serology; predominantly axonal neuropathy on EMG |
| Brainstem vascular malformations | Recurrent infarctions; "flow voids" on MRI; abnormal diffusion MRI or angiography |
| Motor neuron disease | Lower motor neuron signs; abnormal EMGs; cerebral, sensory, or sphincter involvement against this diagnosis |

CT = computed tomography; EMG = electromyography; HIV = human immunodeficiency virus; HTLV-I = human T-cell lymphotropic virus type I.

"Benign MS" is uncommon: Over time, most patients worsen physically or cognitively. After 10 years of disease, about one-third of patients are severely disabled and require institutional care. Another third have significant disability but can be partially employed and maintain social functions. The remaining third have mild or no handicaps.

Multiple sclerosis follows a progressive course in most patients. Seventy percent of persons cannot work full-time. Recent studies indicate that brain atrophy is frequent and progressive in MS patients. Mortality is mostly linked to disability, not exacerbations. Life expectancy is reduced approximately 7 years, with deaths related to aspiration pneumonia, decubiti, urosepsis, or suicide.

Some postulated favorable prognostic signs include:
- Female sex
- Age at onset less than 40 years
- Sensory exacerbations
- Infrequent exacerbations during the first 2 years
- Good response to corticosteroids
- Nonconfluent, discrete "salt-and-pepper" T2 lesions on brain MRI

Unfavorable signs include:
- Male sex
- Older age at onset
- Early and significant cerebellar or pyramidal dysfunction
- Early dementia
- Frequent disabling attacks at onset
- Confluent, widespread lesions on brain MRI, with brainstem and cerebellar involvement

## TREATMENT

**PEARL: No current treatment is proved to arrest the natural history of MS.**

## Primary Treatment

*CONTROVERSY: Individuals with an isolated demyelinating episode such as optic neuritis, brainstem dysfunction, or myelitis, and MRI evidence of other clinically silent lesions, are commonly treated with a course of intravenous methylprednisolone, followed by a rapid oral taper of prednisone. This treatment may postpone the time to onset of clinically definite MS, but its effectiveness has not been proved in prospective studies. Whether treatment with an immunomodulating agent such as beta-interferon in such situations can delay or prevent the onset of clinically definite MS is under active study.*

Most exacerbations are mild and do not require treatment. Corticosteroids are a mainstay of therapy; their main benefit is accelerating recovery from the exacerbation but they are not proved to impede long-term disability. Severe exacerbations causing major impairments of function are often treated with i.v. methylprednisolone 500 to 1000 mg daily for 3 to 5 days, with or without rapid oral prednisone taper (1 mg/kg, tapered over 7 to 10 days). Moderate exacerbations may improve after brief pulses of oral corticosteroids. When starting corticosteroids, potential short-term adverse effects (depression, weight gain, psychosis) and long-term adverse effects (osteoporosis, avascular necrosis) should be discussed and documented.

**Beta-interferons** are immunomodulators that reduce the frequency, severity, and duration of exacerbations in MS. Possible mechanisms include (1) antagonism of gamma-interferon, (2) inhibition of matrix metalloproteinases, (3) reduction of tumor necrosis factor, (4) enhancement of suppressor cell function, (5) enhancement of interleukin-4 and interleukin-10, and (6) enhancement of transforming growth factor beta. On T2-

weighted MRI, beta-interferons reduce the lesion load, and on T1-weighted images, they inhibit gadolinium enhancement. Side effects of interferons are common and consist of a flulike syndrome, injection-site reactions (when given subcutaneously), fever, and myalgias. These adverse effects dwindle over time. Beta-interferons may induce neutralizing antibodies that impair their positive effects.

**Copolymer-1,** a protein composed of the major amino acids in myelin basic protein as a random polymer, is given by subcutaneous injection daily. Copolymer-1 decreases exacerbations in MS but has no persuasive impact on sustained disability.

**PEARL: Immunomodulatory agents alter the natural history of MS and likely work best when initiated early and continued regularly.**

*CONTROVERSY: Criteria for initiating immunomodulating agents in MS are evolving. Suggested useful criteria are*
- *Definite MS (clinical or lab supported)*
- *Frequent or severe attacks*
- *Residual neurologic deficits*
- *Adverse prognosis on MRI*

Patients with significant breakthrough exacerbations or secondary progression while taking immunomodulating agents are treated with intravenous immunoglobulin G and immunosuppressants such as cyclophosphamide, azathioprine, cyclosporine, methotrexate, cladribine, total lymphoid irradiation, or mitoxantrone. Prospective, blinded, controlled trials of these agents have shown modest benefits or conflicting outcomes. Complications include hypersensitivity, infection, bone marrow suppression, liver dysfunction, sterility, and carcinogenesis.

## Secondary Treatment

Secondary treatments in MS ameliorate symptoms. Physical therapy has proved useful in MS. A physical therapist can help to develop and reinforce regular exercise; prevent deconditioning, contractures, and decubiti; identify suitable prosthetic and orthotic devices; and teach safe and efficient gait patterns and transfers.

*Fatigue* is the most pervasive and disabling symptom of MS. It should be differentiated from spasticity, weakness, medication adverse effects, medical illness or infection, and depression. Nonpharmacologic management includes scheduled resting, daytime naps, and exercising in brief intervals only to subfatigue levels. Swimming is the ideal exercise. Amantadine at doses of 100 to 200 mg/day can reduce fatigue. Pemoline (18.75 to 75 mg/day or higher) is an alternative. Other agents, not proved in controlled trials, include methylphenidate, selegiline, selective serotonin-reuptake inhibitors (fluoxetine, sertraline, paroxetine), venlafaxine, and modafenil.

*Spasticity* is common and most disabling when accompanied by painful flexor or extensor spasms. Adductor spasticity interferes with perineal hygiene, transfers, and catheter care. Occult or overt urinary tract infections or fecal impaction may provoke a sudden increase in spasticity. Baclofen, tizanidine, clonidine, benzodiazepines, dantrolene, and cyclobenzaprine help reduce spasticity. The combination of tizanidine (12 to 16 mg/day in divided doses) and baclofen is particularly useful. In carefully selected patients, the intrathecal baclofen pump may control symptomatic spasticity refractory to oral agents.

*Depression* is common in MS. Many patients benefit from antidepressants that exploit the side effect profile (e.g., a more sedating agent for insomnia). Selective serotonin-reuptake inhibitors are activating and cause less constipation and urinary retention than tricyclics. Supportive psychotherapy and group counseling are beneficial.

**Bladder dysfunction** involves a failure to store or to empty urine, or both. Urodynamics studies show three bladder patterns: hyperreflexia, detrusor sphincter dyssynergia, and flaccidity. An initial approach is to measure postvoid residuals. A volume of urine greater than 100 mL suggests a flaccid bladder, best managed by intermittent self-catheterization. Urinary tract infection caused by self-catheterization is uncommon. For patients with persistent symptoms or recurrent urinary tract infections after initial therapy, a complete urologic work-up is recommended. Bladder hyperreflexia is managed by judicious use of anticholinergics, whereas detrusor-sphincter dyssynergia calls for anticholinergics, alpha-blockade, and self-catheterization. Tolteridine, oxybutinin, propantheline, and low doses of tricyclics are effective. Some cases of detrusor-sphincter dyssynergia respond to terazosin or tamsulosin. Frequent nocturia may be disabling, from sleep disruption. Patients with nocturia can catheterize before bedtime and then inhibit bladder function with anticholinergics. Alternatively, desmopressin (10 to 20 μg intranasally at sleep) produces nocturnal antidiuresis. Patients with sudden changes in bladder function should have urinalysis and culture. Indwelling urinary catheters increase the risk of infection and sphincter damage; they should be avoided. A suprapubic cystostomy is preferable in bed-bound patients.

*Constipation* may be worsened by medications (e.g., anticholinergics). Hydration, stool softeners, bowel stimulants, and osmotic agents may be tried. Suppositories and enemas are needed in more severe cases.

*Sexual dysfunction* in men is managed by counseling about alternative techniques, sildenafil citrate (Viagra 25 to 100 mg 1 hour prior to coitus), intracavernosal injections of papaverine or prostaglandin, intraurethral prostaglandin, vacuum pumps, or (rarely) penile implants. Women benefit from using vibrators, copious lubrication, and counseling in alternative techniques to promote arousal and orgasm.

*Pain* is frequent in MS and not clearly related to duration of disease or disability. Trigeminal neuralgia and dysesthetic pain in the limbs are attributed to demyelination of the root entry zone in the cranial nerves or dorsal horns. Neuropathic pain can usually be managed with anticonvulsants (e.g., gabapentin, carbamazepine, topiramate), baclofen, and tricyclic antidepressants. Some patients require these in combination with opioids. Patients with refractory trigeminal neuralgia are candidates for radiofrequency coagulation or gamma-knife radiation of the gasserian ganglion. Annoying limb paresthesias may respond to tricyclics and gabapentin. Lumbar spondylosis causing back pain often complicates MS of long duration in older patients.

*Sleep disturbances* are common. Their differential diagnoses include frequent nocturia, depression, painful limb spasms, anxiety, and restless leg syndrome.

*Paroxysmal symptoms* can present as tonic, seizurelike motor events with paroxysmal posturing, dystonia, or dysarthria. These episodes respond to anticonvulsants or acetazolamide. About 5% of MS patients develop epilepsy.

## Tertiary Treatment

Tertiary treatment prevents long-term complications. Vitamin C (1 g qid) and cranberry juice acidify the urine and prevent recurrent urinary tract infections. Routine surveillance with urinalysis and culture prevents recurrent cystitis and pyelonephritis. Frequent turning and positioning help to prevent decubiti and osteomyelitis. Prophylaxis with vitamin D, calcium supplements, and estrogen replacement (when indicated) may retard osteoporosis, a pervasive complication in MS. Also useful in minimizing osteoporosis are limitations on smoking, ethanol consumption, and the use of corticosteroids. Regular exercise (e.g., swimming) and physical therapy promote cardiovascular health, reduce spasticity and pain, and improve psychological well-being.

The impact of the disease on the patient's lifestyle, family, and community relationships must be explored. Ambulation aids, home alterations, and motor vehicle alterations may improve quality of life. Emotional support and constant encouragement, with a flexible doctor-patient relationship, are crucial elements in holistic management.

# 12

CHAPTER

# Sleep Disorders

**Sleep** is a complex, active state with cyclic changes of brain activity. There are two major sleep periods: rapid eye movement (REM) and nonrapid eye movement (non-REM). Non-REM is divided into a range of four stages, from 1 (drowsiness) to 4 (deep sleep). Most dreams occur during REM sleep, when the electroencephalogram becomes desynchronized (similar to wakefulness), and there is greater irregularity in heart and respiratory rates. Elderly subjects have much less stage 4 non-REM sleep, more frequent awakenings, and less total sleep time.

Sleep disorders cause abnormalities in sleep "architecture" and include insomnia, abnormal behavior such as restless legs, sleep breathing disorders, and excessive daytime somnolence. Sleep disorders mainly seen during non-REM sleep in children (e.g., enuresis, or bedwetting; somnambulism; and night terrors) are not covered here.

Patients should routinely be questioned about their sleep:

- Are there difficulties with falling asleep, staying asleep, or awakening early?
- Does the patient feel refreshed after a night's sleep?

- Does the patient feel tired during the day or suffer from sleep attacks?
- Does the patient's bed partner notice snoring, apneas, or abnormal movements?
- Does the patient have associated daytime symptoms such as paresthesias, sleep paralysis, cataplexy, or hallucinations on falling asleep or awakening?

The diagnosis of sleep disorders is often made with polysomnography. During a night's sleep, several physiologic measures typically are recorded: electromyogram of chin, leg, and respiratory muscles; electrocardiogram; electro-oculogram; respiratory rate and nasal air flow; oxygen saturation; and electroencephalogram. Abnormalities in sleep duration, architecture, arousals, respiration, and movement can be identified, as well as **parasomnias** (abnormal activities during sleep) and seizures.

## RESTLESS LEGS SYNDROME AND PERIODIC MOVEMENTS OF SLEEP

*Restless legs syndrome* and *periodic movements of sleep* are disorders of obscure origin that are more common and more severe in older individuals. Most patients with restless legs syndrome have periodic movements during sleep (see below). **Restless legs syndrome** is characterized by deep paresthesias and crawling sensations of the calves and legs during inactive waking rest periods, while seated or recumbent. Symptoms may be worse at night. Leg movement relieves the unpleasant sensations. The disorder is usually lifelong, and family history is often positive. The results of lab studies are normal except for polysomnography, which usually reveals periodic leg movements. Carbamazepine, levodopa, clonazepam, and opioids (especially oxycodone) are temporarily effective, but tolerance often develops; alternating medications may be useful. Transcutaneous electrical nerve stimulation may help.

**Periodic leg movements of sleep** are stereotyped movements in a prolonged series. Dorsiflexion of the ankle and small toes with or without the great toe and flexion of the knee and hip are most common. The movements, which are slower than myoclonic jerks, are often terminated by a violent other jerk. Some patients complain about poor sleep and excessive daytime somnolence; for others, only the bed partner complains. The disorder is often chronic. Surface electromyography of the anterior tibial muscles is diagnostic. Clonazepam is the treatment of choice; baclofen, imipramine, and opioids can be effective.

## RAPID EYE MOVEMENT BEHAVIORAL DISORDER

Patients who have **REM behavioral disorders** do not have the muscle atonia normally present during REM sleep, and they display elaborate and often violent motor activity usually associated with dreaming. The disorder is diagnosed if the patient has one of the following: dream mentation with harmful or potentially harmful sleep behavior, sleep behavior disrupting sleep continuity, or "acted-out" dreams. Patients have intermittently increased tone of the submental muscles during REM sleep, and most exhibit periodic leg movements during sleep. Clonazepam is often effective.

# EXCESSIVE DAYTIME SOMNOLENCE

Excessive daytime sleepiness and irresistible sleep attacks, usually lasting less than 20 minutes, are the hallmarks of **narcolepsy.** The disorder usually begins before age 25 and is lifelong. Most patients have human leukocyte antigen (HLA)–type DR2 or DQw1. Sleep attacks usually occur during boring or quiet periods (watching TV, reading) but may occur while driving or during stimulating activities.

Auxiliary symptoms include cataplexy (75% of patients), sleep paralysis (35%), and hypnogogic hallucinations (35%). **Cataplexy** is a brief (seconds to 2 minutes), sudden loss of muscle control with preserved consciousness, which may cause a fall, buckling of the knees, or head nod. Attacks are often precipitated by strong emotion (hearty laughter, surprise, crying). **Sleep paralysis** (temporary loss of muscle tone; the patient is awake but unable to move) and **hypnagogic hallucinations** (vivid auditory, visual, vestibular, or somatosensory phenomena that occur while falling asleep) happen during the transition from wakefulness to sleep. Hallucinations also can occur on awakening **(hypnopompic hallucinations).**

Multiple sleep latency tests to detect short sleep latency or sleep-onset REM periods and HLA testing help to establish the diagnosis. Methylphenidate (Ritalin) and dextroamphetamine (Dexedrine) are the treatments of choice for sleep attacks. Imipramine, protryptyline, and other tricyclic antidepressants are helpful for cataplexy but have no effect on sleep attacks.

# SLEEP BREATHING DISORDER

**Sleep apnea syndrome** is defined by cessation of breathing lasting 10 seconds or more and occurring more than 30 times per night. The degree of nocturnal oxygen desaturation and daytime symptoms (excessive sleepiness, sleep attacks, morning headache) and nocturnal signs (snoring, awakenings) are critical features. Sleep apnea is most common in men and patients with obesity and hypertension.

Apneas are classified as *central, obstructive* (peripheral), or *mixed*. In **central apneas,** thoracic and abdominal respiratory muscles are inactive. Snoring is rare but bed partners report cessation of breathing during sleep. Patients experience excessive daytime sleepiness and insomnia.

In **obstructive apneas,** which are much more common than central types, respiratory muscles are active but respiration is impaired by upper airway blockade. Patients have a history of snoring and gasping sounds, nocturnal breath cessations and arousals, excessive nocturnal movements and sweating, morning headache, impaired concentration and cognition, excessive daytime sleepiness and sleep attacks, impotence, and hypertension.

Management of obstructive sleep apnea includes weight loss, medroxyprogesterone or acetazolamide, nasal continuous positive airway pressure, uvulopalatopharyngoplasty to enlarge the pharyngeal airspace, or tracheostomy for severe cases.

# 13
## CHAPTER

# *Conversion Disorder and Malingering*

## DEFINITIONS

**Conversion disorder** is characterized by symptoms or signs that suggest neurologic or medical disorders but actually result from psychological factors. In contrast, **malingering** is the intentional (conscious) production of symptoms. Conversion disorder and malingering can present in any medical setting, but they occur more often in inpatient and emergency wards than in outpatient, medical, surgical, psychiatric, or neurologic settings. The related **somatization disorder,** characterized by a pattern of recurring, nonintentional, multiple somatic complaints that are clinically significant (e.g., requiring medications or impairing function), is more often seen in the outpatient setting.

## PATHOGENESIS

Primary or secondary gain often underlies conversion symptoms. In **primary gain,** an internal conflict or need is suppressed by the symptom. In **secondary gain,** the symptom allows the patient to receive support or avoid unpleasant situations.

# DIAGNOSIS

**PEARL: Diagnosis of conversion disorder requires a high index of suspicion.** Misdiagnosis of conversion disorders as an organic syndrome and misdiagnosis of organic disorders as conversion symptoms are common. Many patients diagnosed with conversion are later found to have neurologic disorders such as multiple sclerosis or lupus. **PEARL: Conversion and organic disorders often co-exist.**

Diagnosis is often difficult. In addition to excluding neurologic or medical disorders, you should look for positive evidence of psychological factors and for features that are inconsistent with principles of neuroanatomy or physiology. Conversion disorder is not diagnosed if symptoms are explained by other psychiatric disorders (e.g., schizophrenia) or result from substance abuse or culturally sanctioned behaviors.

Conversion disorder most often manifests neurologic signs or symptoms, including:

- Motor symptoms (paralysis, seizures, contractures or spasms, tremor, speech disorders, or mutism)
- Sensory symptoms (loss of tactile or visual sensation)
- Other neurologic features (pain, gait disorders such as reeling unsteadiness or astasia-abasia [see Chapter 10], amnesia, coma)

*Malingering* is associated with many neurologic symptoms, most often pain or weakness. Suspect it when:

- Symptoms can provide financial gain.

- Patients have seen numerous physicians and are unhappy with prior care.
- Patients are uncooperative during evaluation and noncompliant with treatment.
- Antisocial personality disorder is present.

## EXAM

Conversion symptoms often fluctuate and have features that follow "lay" concepts of illness, *not* anatomic and physiologic principles. It may help to observe patients when they believe they are unobserved; patients complaining of severe weakness or pain sometimes show no evidence of such problems when unobserved. Nevertheless, differentiating symptoms of conversion or malingering from organic disease can be difficult. The following guidelines may be helpful.

### Paralysis

Note the patient's cooperation and effort. With urging, the patient often makes a brief but maximal effort followed by a weak or absent effort (i.e., "give-way" weakness). When asked to make a movement, the patient may make the opposite movement (contract antagonists) or make a series of partial, irregular contractions (e.g., the "milk maid sign" of serial contraction and relaxation when asked to squeeze fingers). Some helpful tests follow:

1. When testing biceps, triceps, or brachioradialis, suddenly shift from resisting to assisting the muscle, and the arm will return to the original position due to the strength of the antagonist.
2. Elevate the patient's arms and quickly release support; note a momentary ability to hold the arms up before they fall.

3. Ask the patient to raise his or her normal leg while supine. The examiner's hand can detect contraction of the "paralyzed" hamstrings by holding a hand under the "weak" leg (Hoover sign).
4. In the case of a weak leg, note a lack of circumduction (present with upper motor neuron lesions) or the presence of dragging the "dead" leg.

## Sensory Loss

Sensory findings in conversion fluctuate with suggestion and repeated exam. There is a tendency to involve all modalities equally, and to follow sharp anatomic boundaries such as the midline or wrist, in contrast to the sensory gradient seen with organic lesions.

Helpful tests to detect functional sensory loss include:

1. *Forced-choice paradigm:* The patient closes his eyes and is informed that you may or may not touch him. He should answer "yes" [I am being touched] or "no," even if it is a guess. Repeat 40 to 50 stimuli in the "anesthetic" area. Patients with conversion often "guess wrong" more than 60% of the time, defying probability.
2. Apply vibration to an area that the patient says is insensitive, but where bone conduction would transmit sensation to a normal area (e.g., on forehead, clavicle), allowing it to be felt. Patient denies feeling vibration.

## TESTING

The evaluation of conversion disorder and malingering often requires noninvasive studies to exclude atypical forms of organic disease. For example, a patient with conversion paraparesis may require evaluation with spinal x-ray, magnetic resonance imaging, and electromyography to exclude a tumor or neuropathic disorder.

## PROGNOSIS AND TREATMENT

The prognosis for conversion disorder varies. The shorter the duration of symptoms, the better the outcome. Psychiatric consultation is important. Identify underlying causes such as sexual abuse, because counseling or therapy can benefit many patients.

# 3
### PART

# *Emergent and Inpatient Neurologic Problems*

# *14*

## CHAPTER

# *Visual Loss and Double Vision*

Typically you will see patients with visual loss and double vision **(diplopia)** urgently in the office or emergency room. **PEARL: The disorders in this chapter require urgent testing, such as imaging or ophthalmologic evaluation, and immediate institution of treatment.**

## VISUAL LOSS

When you are confronted with a patient with visual loss, the first step is to describe the distribution of the deficit to identify its location in the nervous system. From the history and physical exam, the neurologist will try to classify visual loss as originating in one of the following areas:
- Orbit or retina
- Optic nerve
- Chiasm
- Visual radiations
- Occipital cortex

The onset, course, and nature of symptoms help

to establish the etiology. Acute visual loss is usually vascular (stroke, temporal arteritis), whereas subacute or chronic loss is often due to multiple sclerosis or tumor.

Localization of visual deficits depends on defining the deficit or the "field cut" in each eye, testing visual acuity, observing the pupillary light reflex, and examining the fundus. You should also consider associated ophthalmologic and neurologic findings. Figure 14–1 shows various visual field deficits and the commonly encountered sites of disease producing each type. The pupillary light reflex is usually most impaired with optic nerve lesions, but it may be impaired by lesions of the chiasm or optic tract. Optic atrophy (pale disk with thin, sparse blood vessels) may follow chronic lesions of the optic nerve, chiasmal tract and optic tract, or geniculate body.

*Hallucinations* may occur with visual loss and be **simple** (spots of light, color, geometric forms) or **complex** (faces). Simple hallucinations occur with visual system lesions in locations from the retina to the calcarine cortex. Complex forms usually occur with destructive or irritative lesions of visual association or limbic areas. Such lesions may also produce **illusions,** or images that may be altered in size **(macropsia, micropsia),** position (near or far **[telopsia]**), shape **(metamorphopsia),** movement, color, or depth of field.

*Retinal lesions* cause monocular visual loss (**amaurosis** [see Fig. 14–1, A]). Visual illusions or simple hallucinations may occur, and visual acuity is impaired if the macula is involved. The fundus is often abnormal, but the pupillary light reflex is usually normal. Perception of blue stimuli is most affected. For all other lesion sites, red stimuli are usually the most affected. Common disorders include carotid artery disease and temporal arteritis. Evaluation and treatment are discussed in other chapters.

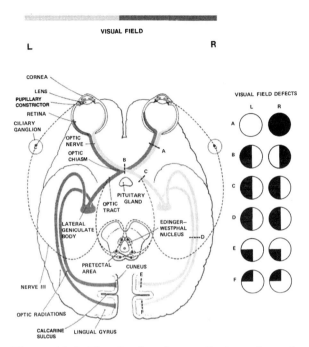

**Figure 14–1.** The visual pathways. Lesions along the pathway from the eye to the visual cortex (lesions A through F) result in defects in the visual fields, which are shown as black areas on the corresponding visual field diagrams. The pathway through the pretectum and cranial nerve III, which mediates reflex constriction of the pupil in response to light, is also shown. (Adapted from Gilman S, and Newman SW: Manter and Gatz's Essentials of Clinical Neuroanatomy and Neurophysiology, ed. 9. F. A. Davis, Philadelphia, 1996, p. 183, with permission.)

*Optic nerve lesions* also cause monocular visual loss. A complete lesion causes blindness. Visual acuity is decreased, and gaze-evoked hallucinations of lights **(phosphenes)** or blindness can occur. Acutely, the fundus may reveal papilledema (swelling and hyperemia of the disk, blurring of the disk margin, and venous distension, some-

times with exudates and hemorrhage). Chronic
lesions produce optic atrophy. The *Marcus Gunn
phenomenon* (afferent pupillary defect) occurs
when light is quickly flashed from the normal
to the impaired eye. The impaired pupil dilates
if there are unilateral or asymmetrical lesions.
Causes include optic neuritis, tumor, or trauma.
These patients need urgent orbital imaging by
computed tomography (CT) or magnetic resonance imaging (MRI).

*Chiasmal lesions* damage crossing fibers from
the nasal portion of each retina. They cause a
bitemporal field cut (see Fig. 14–1, B) and mildly
impaired visual acuity. Pituitary tumors can compress the chiasm, which is slightly above and be-
hind the pituitary gland. Meningiomas, chordomas, and carotid aneurysms also cause chiasmal
compression. These patients need urgent imaging
of the brain by CT or MRI, with attention to the
pituitary area.

*Optic tract lesions* and *lateral geniculate lesions*
cause homonymous hemianopia (see Fig. 14–1,
C), which is often incongruous (the field defect is
asymmetrical from eye to eye). It may be associated with mild contralateral pyramidal (upper
motor neuron) signs from involvement of the
cerebral peduncle. Visual acuity is normal. The
pupillary light reflex may be impaired with optic
tract lesions. Causes include pituitary tumors,
craniopharyngiomas, chordomas, meningiomas,
and stroke. These patients need urgent brain imaging by MRI.

Lesions of the *optic radiations* and *calcarine
cortex* cause homonymous hemianopia (see Fig.
14–1, D) contralateral to the side of the lesion,
with sparing of central vision (macular sparing).
Restricted optic tract lesions can cause a *quadrantanopia:*

• With parietal lesions, the visual loss affects

only the inferior half of the affected side (the inferior "quadrant" [see Fig. 14–1, E]).

- With temporal lesions, vision is lost in the superior portion of the affected field (see Fig. 14–1, F).

Restricted calcarine cortex lesions also can cause a quadrantanopia (inferior with superior lesions and superior with inferior lesions). With calcarine cortex lesions, moving stimuli are perceived better than stationary ones. **PEARL: Patients who have disease in the parietal and temporal lobes commonly have associated sensorimotor and language or spatial disturbances. Those with occipital cortex disease typically do not.**

Causes of lesions in the optic radiations or calcarine cortex include stroke, tumor, trauma, and demyelination. These patients need urgent brain imaging by CT or MRI.

## DOUBLE VISION

Double vision (diplopia) always starts suddenly, as soon as disease prevents the eyes from remaining conjugate. Recent onset of diplopia virtually always requires urgent or emergent evaluation. In the history, inquire about the horizontal or vertical separation of objects. This helps to identify the specific muscles involved.

Physical exam confirms the pattern of involvement. Observe eye movement in all directions (Fig. 14–2). **PEARL: Weakness of one extraocular muscle will produce the greatest degree of diplopia when gaze is directed into the field where that muscle moves the eye. The abnormal eye can be directly observed. When the abnormality is subtle, the abnormal eye can be identified by covering the eyes one at a time. Covering the abnormal eye causes the image farthest from the**

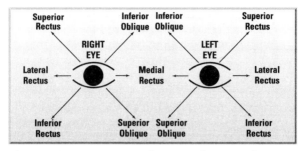

**Figure 14–2.** Directions of action of extraocular muscles. (From Józefowicz RF and Holloway RG, Case Studies in Neuroscience, Philadelphia, F. A. Davis, 1999, p 55, with permission.)

**midline to disappear.** If the eyes seem normal despite careful exam, ask the patient to maintain upgaze for 2 to 3 minutes in an effort to precipitate diplopia or ptosis, as in neuromuscular junction disease (see Chapter 15). Also inquire whether fatigue precipitates symptoms and rest relieves them; this pattern suggests a neuromuscular junction disease. Observe the patient for ptosis and pupillary abnormalities, which are seen with third nerve palsy. **Exophthalmos** (protrusion of one or both eyes) may cause ophthalmoplegia. Common causes of exophthalmos include thyroid disease, tumor, inflammation, cavernous sinus thrombosis, and fistula.

## Diplopia Caused by Unilateral Lesions

Common causes of double vision are isolated unilateral lesions of cranial nerves III, IV, or VI (Table 14–1). **PEARL: Only third and fourth nerve lesions may be associated with vertical diplopia, and sixth nerve lesions produce only horizontal diplopia.** Third nerve lesions may also cause horizontal diplopia.

Third nerve lesions are typically microvascular,

**Table 14–1. CRANIAL NERVE LESIONS
CAUSING DOUBLE VISION**

| Affected Cranial Nerve | Impairment and Associated Signs | Most Frequent Causes |
|---|---|---|
| III | Any combination of impaired adduction, elevation, or depression of the eye (vertical or horizontal diplopia) | Microvascular disorders Aneurysm |
| | Possible pupillary enlargement and ptosis | |
| IV | Impaired depression of the eye in adducted position (vertical diplopia) | Head trauma |
| VI | Impaired abduction of the eye (horizontal diplopia) | Raised intracranial pressure |

but aneurysm must be ruled out. **PEARL: Every patient presenting with third nerve disease, especially if it affects the pupillary light reflex, should be considered for emergency evaluation for aneurysm and subarachnoid hemorrhage.** Patients with diabetes mellitus may develop a pupil-sparing third nerve palsy of sudden onset. An enlarging or hemorrhaging posterior communicating artery aneurysm may present in the same way; the pupil is spared for the first several days but is almost always involved eventually. Patients with diabetic third nerve palsy are observed for a time and often improve. If an aneurysm is suspected, the patient undergoes CT scanning, lumbar puncture, and four-vessel angiography.

Fourth nerve lesions are often due to head trauma and sixth nerve lesions to raised intracranial pressure. Combination lesions should prompt a search for cavernous sinus disease. *Internuclear ophthalmoplegia* is caused by a lesion of the medial longitudinal fasciculus between the pons and midbrain. The ipsilateral eye fails to adduct on lateral gaze to the other side; the abducting eye shows more prominent nystagmus. Convergence is normal. Causes are multiple sclerosis and vascular disease.

## Diplopia Caused by Bilateral Lesions

Bilateral oculomotor lesions occur with:
- *Myasthenia gravis:* This immunologic disorder of the neuromuscular junction may mimic nerve or brainstem lesions. The pupils are not involved. Persistent muscle use often worsens the deficit.
- *Botulism:* The toxin interferes with presynaptic acetylcholine release at the neuromuscular junction. Symptoms begin 12 to 36 hours after ingestion. Blurred and double vision usually appears first. The pupils are affected but there is no fever and the number of lymphocytes in the cerebrospinal fluid is not increased.
- *Miller-Fisher syndrome:* This variant of acute inflammatory demyelinating polyneuropathy causes bilateral ophthalmoplegia (see Chapter 15). The pupils are affected.
- *Parinaud's syndrome*: This is caused by mass lesions (such as pineal tumors) exerting pressure on the tectum and superior colliculi. Upgaze is more affected by paralysis than downgaze. **Mydriasis** (large pupils), impaired convergence, and loss of pupillary light reflex occur with this syndrome.

Other causes of bilateral oculomotor lesions are meningitis (bacterial or carcinomatous), Wernicke's encephalopathy (from thiamine deficiency), and drugs (antiepileptic drug toxicity).

# 15
## CHAPTER

# *Weakness*

You may encounter patients with weakness in any clinical setting. The degree and distribution of weakness and its onset may differ by setting, however. Patients with sudden weakness or with difficulty walking or breathing are typically evaluated in urgent settings.

Weakness may be central (from disease of the central nervous system) or peripheral. The distinction is made by history and physical exam. Hemibody weakness or isolated limb weakness associated with spasticity and hyperreflexia is due to brain or spinal cord disease such as stroke, tumor, or multiple sclerosis. These disorders are discussed elsewhere. Here we focus on weakness caused by peripheral neuromuscular disorders. This kind of weakness is often associated with hypotonia, areflexia, atrophy, or fasciculations.

Weakness is common with peripheral neuropathy, neuromuscular junction disease, muscle disease, and motor neuron disease. You can identify and distinguish between these various types through the patient's history and physical exam. If necessary, electromyography (EMG) and nerve conduction velocity (NCV) testing are performed to help establish the diagnosis (Table 15–1).

**Table 15–1. CHARACTERISTIC FEATURES OF NEUROMUSCULAR DISORDERS**

| Feature | Nerve Diseases | Neuromuscular Junction Disease | Muscle Disease |
|---------|----------------|-------------------------------|----------------|
| Weakness | Distal | Increased with persistent effort | Proximal |
| Reflexes | Diminished | Normal | Normal or diminished late |
| Sensory loss | Distal | None | None |
| Nerve conduction | Slow or normal | Normal | Normal |
| EMG | Denervation Loss of motor units Increased polyphasia | Decremental repetitive stimulation | Low-amplitude, short-duration potentials |

# PERIPHERAL NEUROPATHY

## Mononeuropathies

**Radial nerve palsy** is an injury to the radial nerve in the spiral groove of the upper arm, resulting from improper and prolonged compression of the upper arm in sleep, intoxicated states, or with anesthesia. Wrist extension is weak, but triceps power is spared. Weakness of the brachioradialis is typical, producing weakness of forearm flexion, and helps to distinguish this disorder from a lower cervical radiculopathy. Sensory loss is mild and usually involves the first dorsal web space. Splints and exercise are the usual treatment, and prognosis is ordinarily very good.

**Bell's palsy** is an idiopathic palsy of the facial nerve that causes facial weakness and may be associated with pain, abnormal taste sensation on the tongue, and an unusual sensitivity to sound. Most patients recover without treatment. Facial nerve conduction studies may be prognostically useful. Bell's palsy is idiopathic, but Lyme disease, diabetes, and sarcoidosis can involve the facial nerve and should be considered. The diagnosis is made clinically, and the patient should be observed for improvement. **PEARL: If the eye cannot be closed, it must be patched to protect against corneal drying and injury.** Steroid therapy instituted within 10 days may shorten the time to recovery.

*CONTROVERSY: Steroid use for Bell's palsy is controversial. The data supporting the use of steroids are not convincing, and the degree of improvement is not enhanced, only the speed of improvement.*

## Polyneuropathies

**Acute idiopathic demyelinating polyneuropathy ([AIDP] Guillain-Barré syndrome)** is characterized by acute to subacute progression (over about 4 weeks) of predominantly motor dysfunction. The patient may have had a respiratory or gastrointestinal (GI) illness just before the onset of weakness. He or she may also have minor sensory dysfunction, and reflexes are usually lost. Some patients report considerable pain, described as "deep pain." The cranial nerves and respiratory musculature are commonly involved, and autonomic instability may occur, particularly in young patients. The diagnosis is established clinically and supported by elevated cerebrospinal fluid (CSF) protein with few cells (albuminocytologic dissociation) and by electrophysiologic studies (electromyography [EMG]). Within the first 1 to 7 days, these test results may be normal. The most frequent early abnormality is a prolonged F response (see "Electromyography" in Chapter 2). AIDP can require emergent neurophysiologic studies. Lyme and human immunodeficiency virus (HIV) titers should be routinely checked. AIDP may be seen in patients infected with HIV who have no other symptoms of that infection.

**PEARL: AIDP is a neurologic emergency requiring hospitalization with careful monitoring of respiratory function.** If vital capacity continually decreases, intubation can be offered on an elective basis. Most patients make an excellent recovery. Plasmapheresis may reduce the duration of assisted ventilation and inability to walk for patients who present within the first 7 to 14 days. Intravenous immune globulin may be used instead of plasmapheresis, but it is difficult to obtain and extremely expensive.

**Chronic idiopathic demyelinating polyneuropathy (CIDP)** is a syndrome similar to the acute disorder, but progressing over at least 2 months. HIV, connective tissue disease, and Lyme disease should be excluded. Treatment is steroids, with plasmapheresis for more acute exacerbations. Plasmapheresis may be used on a repeat basis with mild forms of the disorder, followed by long-term azathioprine therapy. Immune globulin may be used as well.

## NEUROMUSCULAR JUNCTION DISEASE

**Myasthenia gravis** is produced by antibody destruction of the postsynaptic acetylcholine receptor and the nearby membrane. The hallmark is weakness after persistent muscle activity, but weakness may also be constant. Patients may be weak or normal on routine exam. Weakness of the muscles of the upper extremity or extraocular muscles may then be elicited by having the patient maintain activity for several minutes. Approximately one in seven patients have weakness restricted to the ocular muscles; others have either mild or severe generalized dysfunction.

## Diagnostic Testing for Myasthenia Gravis

The diagnosis is clinical and confirmed with an edrophonium (Tensilon) test and repetitive stimulation study on EMG. To perform a Tensilon test, identify an area of objective weakness, most often in the eyelids. (Do not use respiratory dysfunction as a marker.) A crash cart with intubation material should be available. Saline or atropine (0.4 mg) should be injected intravenously as a control, given before the edrophonium; atropine can reverse the muscarinic side effects of the edrophonium. Administer edrophonium 2 mg i.v. push; if that is well tolerated, give 3 mg and then 5 mg (to a 10-mg total). Improved neurologic function suggests myasthenia gravis. Side effects such as excessive salivation, lacrimation, urination, and diarrhea, as well as hypotension and bradycardia, are all possible. If the patient has established myasthenia and is already being treated with anticholinesterase medications, any increase of weakness suggests that reduction of the dosage is indicated.

At another time, perform repetitive stimulation by EMG (three stimuli per second) to identify decremental conduction. Single-fiber EMG is a sensitive but nonspecific test that may reveal increased jitter consistent with neuromuscular junction disease. Patients should be tested for acetylcholine receptor antibodies, but not all patients with the disease are positive for these antibodies. A computed tomography scan of the mediastinum should be performed to identify thymus hyperplasia or thymoma, both of which are sometimes seen in patients with myasthenia.

## Treatment of Myasthenia Gravis

Patients with systemic myasthenia should be admitted to the hospital when treatment is first instituted, unless their symptoms are extremely mild. They should avoid drugs that precipitate weakness, such as sedatives, aminoglycosides, propranolol, and many others. Hyperthyroidism should be excluded with appropriate serum testing. Those with severe dysfunction should be placed in an intensive care unit or stepdown unit and monitored for respiratory failure. Shortness of breath or a progressively diminishing forced vital capacity calls for elective intubation.

Patients who have generalized disease should be treated with anticholinesterase therapy if they are young (under age 50) and with steroid therapy if they are older. Anticholinesterase therapy typically is not used for older patients, except for brief periods of symptom control, because of potential side effects. Steroid therapy may be associated with initial symptomatic worsening, so it should be started in the hospital. Immune therapy for young patients usually involves thymectomy rather than chronic steroid therapy. Radiation therapy may be used if thymoma is present and removal is incomplete. Prolonged anticholinesterase therapy is not recommended for generalized disease if immune therapy is effective. Acute, severe generalized myasthenia requires hospitalization and plasmapheresis followed by azathioprine therapy for immune suppression.

Patients of any age with isolated ocular myasthenia are usually managed with anticholinesterase medication. Typical starting dose is oral Mestinon (pyridostigmine) 60 mg every 3 to 4 hours, with or without a 180-mg sustained-release dose at night. Steroids may be helpful during exacerbations.

## MUSCLE DISEASE

**Polymyositis** is characterized by subacute and variable proximal muscle weakness and fatigue. One of every three patients has cardiac and pulmonary dysfunction. Typically, the neck and muscles below the neck are involved, but dysphagia is uncommon. The extraocular muscles are typically spared. **Dermatomyositis** is diagnosed if patients have a concomitant erythematous rash. One in five patients with dermatomyositis has a systemic carcinoma. In both disorders, check for elevated levels of creatinine kinase, transaminases, and aldolase. Myoglobinuria occurs in severe cases. Muscle enzyme elevations reflect disease activity; the erythrocyte sedimentation rate does not. EMG reveals myopathic abnormalities. Muscle biopsy confirms the diagnosis, revealing inflammation and necrosis or perifascicular atrophy.

Treatment is steroid therapy at 80 mg/day, reduced slowly over months, eventually to every other day. Patients usually require 24 months of treatment. Methotrexate or azathioprine may be used as steroid-sparing agents. Older patients and those with carcinoma do not respond well to therapy. Beginning treatment before atrophy develops results in a better prognosis. Discontinue immune therapy if the patient does not improve after 2 months. Steroid myopathy, presenting as increased weakness without an increase in muscle enzymes, may develop. If this is clinically suspected, reduce the steroid dose. Physical therapy may be helpful.

**Muscular dystrophy** (Duchenne's, Becker's, facioscapulohumeral, or limb-girdle) is characterized by progressive atrophy and weakness. These are familial disorders, but family history is absent in one-third of patients with the Duchenne type. Most patients with muscular dystrophy survive, but those with Duchenne's dystrophy, which affects only male patients, typically die in the second or third decade from respiratory insufficiency, heart disease, or infection. The cause of Duchenne's dystrophy is absent dystrophin in the muscle membrane. Reduced or dysfunctional dystrophin produces Becker's dystrophy. Onset is usually in childhood. Biopsy will exclude the benign nemaline and central-core myopathies. Duchenne's and Becker's dystrophy can be detected by polymerase chain reaction using a restriction fragment length polymorphism (RFLP) linkage analysis. Dystrophin in a muscle sample may also be tested. Carriers may have elevated creatinine kinase levels. These patients need aggressive physical and respiratory therapy. They should avoid bed rest because it increases weakness. Parents and carriers should receive genetic counseling. Some mothers choose to abort male fetuses with the Duchenne gene.

*Myotonic dystrophy* may occur anywhere from childhood to late adulthood, but the symptoms are often denied by the patient. This disorder is inherited via chromosome 19 in an autosomal dominant pattern. Untreatable weakness, usually distal, is the major symptom. Patients present with ptosis, an unusual deformity of the mouth ("fish mouth"), distal upper extremity atrophy, myotonia manifested as impaired hand relaxation, percussion myotonia, cataracts, diminished IQ (static), hypogonadism, esophageal dysfunction, and sleep apnea. EMG reveals myotonic responses (with a characteristic sound likened to an old "dive bomber," heard as the signals are visualized by the EMG device) and myopathic features (see Chapter 2). The myotonia may be treatable with phenytoin or procainamide. Respiratory and speech therapy may be used for patients with pulmonary and swallowing dysfunction.

Eating undercooked pork may result in infection by *Trichinella spiralis*, a GI parasite. The parasite causing *trichinosis* travels from the blood to muscle, producing GI symptoms, fever, periorbital edema, muscular aches, and generalized weakness. Eosinophilia and muscle biopsy to detect the parasite establish the diagnosis. Prednisone may ameliorate symptoms, but thiabendazole is the definitive treatment.

**Hypokalemic periodic paralysis** is an autosomal dominant disorder that typically occurs in male adolescents or young men, who have sudden attacks of quadriparesis (which spares bulbar and respiratory function) associated with muscle weakness and diminished reflexes. The attacks last hours. Carbohydrate intake, exercise, or cold temperatures may precipitate an attack. Diagnosis is confirmed by reduced potassium levels during an attack and an EMG showing impaired muscle excitability. Patients should be evaluated for hyperthyroidism. An acute attack may be treated with potassium replacement. Chronic potassium replacement, a low-carbohydrate diet, and acetazolamide may be used prophylactically. Patients with thyroid disease only require therapy for the thyroid disorder.

**Hyperkalemic periodic paralysis,** an autosomal dominant disorder, affects male and female patients equally. It typically occurs in childhood with attacks of weakness that last approximately

1 hour. Myotonia may be present during attacks and may be detected on EMG, along with excessively excitable muscles. Because they are brief, acute attacks usually do not need treatment, but they may be aborted by intravenous calcium, glucose, or epinephrine. Acetazolamide can be used as chronic preventive therapy.

## MOTOR NEURON DISEASE

**Amyotrophic lateral sclerosis (ALS)** is the most common form of motor neuron disease and is characterized by progressive loss of upper and lower motor neurons. Other forms of motor neuron disease include **progressive spinal muscular atrophy,** in which only the anterior horn cells are involved, and **primary lateral sclerosis,** an extremely rare variant in which only the corticospinal pathways are affected.

### Signs and Symptoms

Motor neuron disease begins most commonly between ages 40 and 60 and affects men more frequently than women. Weakness begins insidiously in the distal limbs and spreads proximally to involve the trunk and cranial musculature. Patients may initially report cramping, aching, and twitching in limb muscles. An asymmetrical presentation is not unusual. Sphincter and extraocular muscles are not involved. Bulbar symptoms such as progressive dysphagia, impaired chewing, nasal or hoarse speech, and respiratory weakness accompany ALS and often indicate a poor prognosis.

The neurologic exam reveals signs of upper and lower motor neuron deficits. Sensation is normal.

Diffuse fasciculations are characteristic of ALS; scan all body surfaces thoroughly for this sign. Exercise, percussion, and cold temperatures may unmask latent fasciculation. You may observe fasciculations and wasting in the tongue. Distal muscle wasting and weakness are combined with hyperreflexia, spasticity, and Babinski signs. The jaw jerk, snout, and gag reflexes may be abnormally exaggerated. Patients also may show pseudobulbar palsy, with uncontrollable laughing and crying. There are no sensory deficits. Cognition is normal.

## Lab Tests

Laboratory investigation includes EMG, nerve conduction studies, and muscle biopsy. Neurophysiologic studies demonstrate normal nerve conduction with signs of active denervation. Muscle biopsy reveals small angulated fibers with group atrophy. In contrast to myopathies, the serum creatinine kinase level is normal or elevated only slightly. About 5% to 10% of cases of ALS are familial, and these cases have recently been linked to a mutation in the gene for superoxide dismutase.

The approach to the patient with motor neuron disease involves excluding treatable disorders:

- *Hyperthyroidism* can cause a proximal, diffuse weakness and hyperreflexia. Thyroid function test results are abnormal.
- *Heavy metal intoxications* (lead, arsenic, mercury) may present with neuropathic weakness and minimal sensory loss. A 24-hour urine collection and serum levels of heavy metals are diagnostic.
- *Disorders of parathyroid metabolism* causing hypocalcemia or hypercalcemia can produce fasciculation, cramping, twitching, and weakness. Parathyroid hormone and calcium levels help to identify these disorders.

- *Cervical spondylosis* and, rarely, *foramen magnum or cervical tumors* cause fasciculation and atrophy in the upper limbs and pyramidal signs in the lower limbs. Magnetic resonance imaging is usually diagnostic.
- *Plasma-cell dyscrasias (gammopathies)* can be associated with the secretion of immunoglobulins targeted at myelin and axonal components. Electrophysiologic studies may show multifocal motor neuronopathy with conduction block, or chronic demyelinating polyneuropathy. Serum and protein immunoelectrophoresis, bone marrow exam, and antibody titers (for serum antibodies against myelin-associated glycoprotein and $GM_1$ gangliosides) are indicated to exclude this potentially treatable cause.

## Treatment

No completely effective therapy exists for ALS. Patients with spinal muscular atrophy may survive for many years; survival with bulbar disease is about 18 months. Overall, the median life span is about 4 years. Recent clinical trials in ALS have focused on glutamate antagonists, on the presumption that excitatory amino acids play a role in motor neuron demise. A recent trial of riluzole showed only modest benefits in prolonging survival in those with bulbar ALS.

Symptomatic therapies for motor neuron disease are available. Muscle spasms can be relieved by physical therapy with stretching, along with judicious use of baclofen (20 to 80 mg daily in divided doses). A nutritious diet with adequate calories should be maintained and may require placement of a feeding gastrostomy tube to prevent aspiration. Tracheostomy should be considered early on to prevent aspiration and to facilitate suctioning. As respiratory strength declines, the decision to undertake mechanical ventilation at home will involve extensive discussions with the patient and caregivers. The patient's philosophy and personal circumstances should be discussed repeatedly in designing advance directives about intubation, mechanical ventilation, antibiotics, gastrostomy, and resuscitation.

# 16
## CHAPTER

# *Cognitive Disorders*

Acquired brain lesions can impair cognitive functions, including language (**aphasia**), reading (**alexia**), writing (**agraphia**), memory (**amnesia**), performance of learned motor acts (**apraxia**), attention (**inattention, neglect**), and visuospatial functions. Before assessing these disorders, determine handedness. Ninety percent of the population is right-handed; 99% of right-handers have language in the left hemisphere, but only 60% of those who are left-handed. (In 10% of left-handers, language is in the right hemisphere, and in 30% it is bilateral.).

*CONTROVERSY: Are cognitive functions localized? Discrete areas of cerebral cortex have specific connections and perform distinct actions. However, complex functions such as attention and language require the integrated activities of multiple "networked" cortical areas.*

Cognitive disorders are most commonly seen in the inpatient service, especially in patients with strokes or tumors. They are also common in outpatient areas (e.g., patients with dementia, tumor) and in the emergency room (e.g., patients with delirium from metabolic or toxic disorders, stroke, central nervous system [CNS] infection). Most cognitive and behavioral disorders can be recognized from a few simple questions and tests, but they are often missed due to lack of suspicion. Chapter 1 outlines the steps to take in examining these patients.

# APHASIA (ACQUIRED LANGUAGE DISORDER)

*Aphasia* must be distinguished from motor and sensory disorders. Aphasias may be classified and localized by the language exam and associated neuropsychiatric findings. There are eight main types of aphasia (Table 16–1): Broca's, global, and transcortical motor aphasia have nonfluent speech and usually result from frontal lesions; Wernicke's, conduction, anomic, and transcortical sensory aphasia have fluent speech and usually result from temporoparietal lesions.

## Anatomy of Language

There are three principal language areas (Fig. 16–1). *Broca's area* lies in the inferior frontal region and controls the motor programs for spoken and written language. *Wernicke's area* lies in the posterior superior temporal gyrus (adjacent to the auditory association cortex) and mediates language comprehension. The **angular** and **supramarginal gyri** of the *parietal lobe* connect language areas with other cortical areas. Parietal language areas help to mediate reading, writing, and naming. (The temporal lobe is also important in naming.)

## Table 16–1. CLINICAL FEATURES OF CORTICAL APHASIAS

| | NONFLUENT APHASIAS | | | | FLUENT APHASIAS | | | |
|---|---|---|---|---|---|---|---|---|
| | Broca's | Mixed Transcortical | Transcortical Motor | Global | Wernicke's | Conduction | Transcortical Sensory | Anomic |
| **Language Findings** | | | | | | | | |
| Paraphasias | Yes, mild | No | No | No | Yes | Yes | Yes | No |
| Comprehension | ± | – | + | – | – | + | – | + |
| Repetition | – | + | + | – | – | – | + | + |
| Naming | ± | – | ± | – | – | – | – | – |
| Reading comprehension | ± | – | + | – | – | ± | – | + |
| Writing | – | – | – | – | – | – | – | + |

**Associated Neuropsychiatric Findings**

| | | | | | | | | |
|---|---|---|---|---|---|---|---|---|
| Motor | HP | HP | HP | HP | + | + | + | + |
| Somatosensory | ±HS | HS | + | HS | ±HS | ±HS | ±HS | + |
| Visual field | + | HA | + | HA | ±Superior QA | ±HA | HA | + |
| Apraxia | ±Left limbs | No | ±Left limbs | ±Bilateral | No | ±Bilateral | No | No |
| Behavior | Depression | Confusion Apathy | Decreased spontaneity Apathy | Depression | Agitation Confusion Paranoia | ± | Agitation Confusion Paranoia | ± |

− = impaired; + = normal; ± = may be impaired or normal; HA = hemianopia; HP = hemiparesis; HS = hemisensory loss; QA = quadrantanopia.

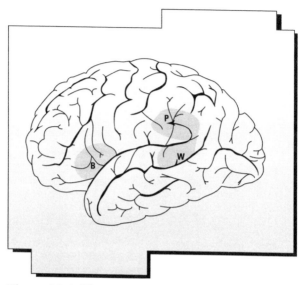

**Figure 16–1.** Three main areas of the brain are critical for language function. Wernicke's area (W) mediates comprehension of spoken language. The parietal language cortex (P) is important for reading, writing, and naming. Broca's area (B) mediates grammar and motor programs for speech. Information is transferred from Wernicke's area to Broca's area along the arcuate fasciculus (arrows).

## Aphasic Disorders

**Broca's aphasia** is characterized by impaired spontaneous speech that is nonfluent, slow, effortful, dysprosodic (abnormal speech rhythm and tone), and telegraphic (using only substantive nouns and verbs). Repetition, naming, reading, and writing are impaired; comprehension is preserved. Right hemiparesis and depression are often present. The most common causes are infarct involving the upper division of the left middle cerebral artery, hemorrhage, tumor, and trauma.

**Wernicke's aphasia** is characterized by fluent speech with normal prosody and frequent paraphasic errors (calling a *shoe* a *too* or a *foot thing*). Comprehension of spoken and written language is impaired, but the impairment may only be evident with specific questioning. Patients may talk excessively and respond somewhat appropriately to questions. Naming, repetition, reading, and writing are impaired. There may be a right visual field cut (complete or affecting the superior quadrant). Psychiatric misdiagnosis can occur because of the preserved fluency and strength as well as agitation, irritability, and suspiciousness. The most common causes are infarct involving the lower division of the left middle cerebral artery, hemorrhage, tumor, or trauma.

**Conduction aphasia** is characterized by a relatively selective impairment of repetition and naming. Speech is fluent with frequent paraphasias, and comprehension is normal or mildly impaired. Reading comprehension is relatively preserved, but reading aloud and writing are impaired. Conduction aphasia results from either disconnection of posterior and anterior language areas (arcuate fasciculus lesion) or damage to the inferior parietal lobe, left auditory cortex, or insula. The most common causes are middle cerebral artery strokes and tumor.

**Anomic aphasia** is characterized by a relatively selective impairment of naming. Patients speak fluently but pause to find words and may circumlocute (i.e., talk around the word they are trying to find), producing "empty speech" with many nonspecific words (*thing, this, you know*). Anomia occurs with lesions in all language areas and may occur with lesions outside the language cortex or with metabolic encephalopathies. The most severe and selective anomias result from dominant temporal lesions.

**Global aphasia** is impairment of all language

functions. Initially, the patient is mute or has effortful, nonfluent speech. Lethargy, decreased attention, right hemiparesis, and hemisensory and visual field deficits often accompany global aphasia. The lesion usually involves left frontal, temporal, and parietal areas and most often results from occlusion of the internal carotid artery or proximal middle cerebral artery, hemorrhage, or tumor.

Other forms of aphasia include *transcortical aphasia*, which results from isolation (not destruction) of language areas and is characterized by preserved repetition. The *motor form* of transcortical aphasia is similar to Broca's aphasia, but with preserved repetition. The lesion is anterior or superior to Broca's area and most often results from infarcts involving the anterior cerebral artery or watershed (anterior cerebral artery and middle cerebral artery), hemorrhage, or tumor. The *sensory form* is similar to Wernicke's aphasia, but with preserved repetition. The lesion is posterior, medial, or superior to Wernicke's area and most often is from infarct involving the middle cerebral artery, posterior cerebral artery, or the watershed between them.

*Subcortical aphasia* can occur with lesions involving the left basal ganglia and anterior limb of the internal capsule or in the left thalamus. These aphasias generally have a better recovery than cortical aphasias.

## Impaired Prosody (Dysprosody)

**Prosody** is variation in the pitch, rhythm, melody, and distribution of stress in speech; it conveys shades of meaning. The right hemisphere modulates **emotional prosody** (tone), and both hemispheres contribute to nonaffective **proposi-

**tional prosody,** such as raising pitch at the end of a sentence to indicate a question. Dysprosody may affect perception and expression. Understanding the emotional prosody and gestures of others also is impaired with right-hemisphere lesions.

## ALEXIA (ACQUIRED READING DISORDER)

An acquired disorder of reading without an acquired disorder of writing, **alexia without agraphia (pure alexia)** results from disconnection of visual input from language areas. Usually, a left posterior cerebral infarct destroys the left visual cortex and posterior corpus callosum, preventing transfer of residual right occipital visual information to left parietal language areas.

**Alexia with agraphia** results from lesions of the angular gyrus. Patients often have a mild fluent aphasia with anomia and paraphasias. Comprehension is preserved. Patients may have features of Gerstmann's syndrome, which is discussed later in this chapter.

## AGRAPHIA (ACQUIRED WRITING DISORDER)

*Agraphia* accompanies all aphasias and helps to distinguish aphasia from motor speech disorders such as dysarthria. Both agraphia and aphasia reflect impaired language function. Agraphia can result from frontal or parietal lesions. *Pure agraphia* is not associated with language, praxis, or motor disorders; it usually occurs with left superior parietal lesions.

# AMNESIA

Brain injury more often affects recent (**short-term**) memory than remote (**long-term**) memory. Impairment affects the learning of new information (**anterograde amnesia**) more than the recall of previously learned information (**retrograde amnesia**).

The medial temporal lobe (hippocampus) and thalamus (dorsomedial nucleus) and their interconnections are the most clinically important structures in the memory network. Left-sided temporal and thalamic lesions selectively impair verbal memory; right-sided lesions impair visual memory. Severe amnesia follows bilateral lesions.

Permanent amnesia is caused by:
- *Medial temporal lesions* that are usually bilateral; they result from encephalitis, tumor, ischemia, or Alzheimer's disease
- *Diencephalic lesions,* which most often occur with stroke or **Korsakoff's disease,** a thiamine deficiency, usually from malnutrition in alcoholics or the seriously ill. Korsakoff's disease may develop after Wernicke's encephalopathy (delirium, ataxia, nystagmus, ophthalmoplegia).

**Transient global amnesia** (**TGA**) is a benign disorder of unknown origin that occurs in those over age 40. It is characterized by confusion, anxiety, and amnesia. The patient repeats questions concerning location, nearby objects, and time but retains personal identity. The duration is 30 minutes to 24 hours, but is usually 2 to 4 hours. Focal neurologic signs are absent during and after the attack. Differential diagnoses include seizures, which usually last less than 5 minutes, and transient ischemic attacks, which are associated with other neurologic abnormalities.

*Conversion disorder* (hysterical) may include amnesia. **PEARL: Being unable to recall personal identity (name or address) while successfully recalling other data (current president, date) very strongly suggests conversion amnesia.** See Chapter 13.

## APRAXIA

**Apraxia,** the inability to perform movements in response to commands, may involve facial muscles, limbs, or truncal muscles. Apraxia does not result from impaired strength, sensation, coordination, comprehension, or attention. Instead, it results from destruction or disconnection of association areas in the dominant hemisphere. Two areas of the left hemisphere control learned motor patterns: one in the frontal lobe controls motor execution and one in the parietal lobe integrates motor sequences with visual and somesthetic information. Apraxia may result from lesions in these areas or from lesions that disconnect these areas from Wernicke's area or motor areas in the left and right hemispheres.

## AGNOSIA

**Agnosia** is impaired recognition despite preserved attention, intelligence, and perception. Agnosias may involve visual, auditory, or tactile modalities. They result from lesions or disconnection of the specific sensory association areas.

## GERSTMANN'S SYNDROME

Damage to the left posteroinferior parietal lobe can cause a tetrad of disorders:
- *Agraphia*
- **Dyscalculia:** an acquired loss of arithmetic skills (mentally or with pen and paper)
- **Finger agnosia:** the inability to recognize, identify, differentiate, and select fingers on one's own or another's hands
- **Right-left disorientation:** the inability to name or point to the left and right sides of body parts or objects

Individual components of this syndrome occur with lesions in other sites.

## NEGLECT SYNDROME

**Unilateral neglect** or inattention is impaired orientation or action toward stimuli from one side, or perception of stimuli from one side, despite preserved movement and sensation. Severity varies from being detectable only with double simultaneous stimulation to profound failure to recognize one's own limb. Unilateral neglect is most common, severe, and persistent with right parietal lesions (usually middle cerebral artery strokes) but also occurs with left parietal, right frontal, and right or left subcortical lesions. The right hemisphere is dominant for attention.

Patients with **anosognosia** fail to recognize their own deficit (e.g., left hemiparesis or cortical blindness [Anton's syndrome]). **Confabulation,** or the "automatic" fabrication or filling in of information, most often when responding to questions, is common in patients with anosognosia, as well as those with Korsakoff's disease and frontal lesions.

# IMPAIRED VISUOSPATIAL ABILITY

The right parietal lobe is dominant for visuospatial perceptual and motor functions (e.g., picturing something in three dimensions or drawing it, orientation of clothing and body parts, geographic orientation). Right parietal lesions, usually from middle cerebral artery strokes, can impair visuospatial abilities and are often accompanied by left-sided neglect.

# 17
## CHAPTER

# Coma and Other States of Impaired Consciousness

The initial approach to the comatose patient is to determine the kind of coma (*structural, metabolic, psychogenic*), based on clinical presentation. Lab tests confirm this categorization, identify the specific cause, and guide therapy (Table 17–1).

## FUNCTIONAL ANATOMY AND EXAM

### Level of Consciousness

Consciousness is maintained by the cerebral hemispheres and the ascending reticular activating system, which projects diffusely to the cerebral cortex from the pons, midbrain, hypothalamus, and thalamus. **PEARL: Damage to both hemispheres or the brainstem impairs consciousness.**

Test the response to specific stimuli, such as calling the patient's name or applying painful fin-

**Table 17–1. CLINICAL AND LABORATORY
FEATURES OF COMA OF
VARYING ETIOLOGIES**

| Coma Type | Focal Signs | Early Course | Diagnostic Tests |
|---|---|---|---|
| Supra-tentorial | Present, often asymmetrical | Progressive deterioration from cortex to brainstem and herniation | CT or MRI |
| Subtentorial | Brainstem signs, extraocular dysfunction | No herniation syndrome | CT and MRI |
| Metabolic | None or symmetrical asterixis, myoclonus, or seizures; pupils usually normal | No herniation syndrome | CT, LP, and testing for systemic disorders |
| Psychogenic | None | No herniation syndrome | CT, LP, and EEG all normal |

LP = lumbar puncture.

gernail pressure. **PEARL: Describe the degree of responsiveness, recording *specific* responses to *specific* stimuli. Coma** refers to a state of eyes-closed unresponsiveness to deep pain. **Stupor** refers to an eyes-closed state during which pain will arouse the patient. **Lethargic** patients respond to voice. Between lethargy and alertness are many degrees of inattentiveness.

## Pupillary Reactivity

**PEARL: Reactive pupils in a comatose patient suggest a metabolic or multifocal etiology,** rather than a single structural cause. The sympathetic nervous system stimulates the pupillodilator muscle and enlarges the pupil (**mydriasis**). The parasympathetic nervous system stimulates the pupillary constrictor and contracts the pupil (**miosis**).

To test the pupillary light reflex, shine a bright light in either eye while the other eye is closed **(direct reflex)**. Then expose each eye to bright light while the other eye is open and checked for the **consensual reflex** of pupillary constriction. Your findings will suggest possible causes of unresponsiveness:

- *Small, reactive pupils:* hypothalamic, bihemispheral, or metabolic dysfunction.
- *Bilateral large, unreactive pupils:* midbrain lesions; similar findings are produced by atropine, scopolamine, and glutethimide.
- *A unilateral large and fixed pupil, with associated ptosis and impaired abduction and elevation of the eye:* oculomotor nerve lesions.
- *Pinpoint reactive pupils:* pontine lesions (damage to descending sympathetic tracts). A magnifying glass may be required to see the response. Similar findings are produced by opioids.

## Extraocular Movements

### *Lateral Gaze*

Pathways from the frontal eye fields descend and cross in the midbrain en route to the pontine lateral gaze center in the reticular formation near the sixth nerve nucleus. The **left parapontine reticular formation** moves the eyes conjugately, horizontally to the left. The **right parapontine reticular formation** moves the eyes conjugately, horizontally to the right. The left hemisphere controls horizontal eye movements to the right, and the right hemisphere controls eye movements to the left.

### Vertical Gaze

Frontal and occipital eye fields send fibers that descend ipsilaterally to the midbrain pretectum, an important area for vertical gaze.

### Corneal Reflexes

The corneal reflex is tested by gently touching the cornea with a wisp of cotton. The reflex involves bilateral eyelid closure and upward eye movement after unilateral corneal stimulation. A normal reflex suggests an intact brainstem from the oculomotor to the facial nerve nuclei.

### Exam

**PEARL: Asymmetrical ocular dysfunction strongly suggests structural coma.** Examine the eyes (pupils and lids) and spontaneous extraocular movements at rest. Shine a light into the eyes from approximately 2 feet away. The light reflecting on the cornea should be in an identical spot in both eyes if they are conjugate. If the lids are held open, they should close very slowly in truly comatose patients. Patients with psychogenic coma cannot mimic this eye closure. Full, spontaneous, bilateral roving eye movements suggest intact horizontal gaze. Table 17–2 summarizes eye movement findings of unresponsive patients.

### Oculocephalic Reflex Testing

If there are no spontaneous roving eye movements, test the *oculocephalic reflex (OCR)*, unless there is a neck injury. Turn the head briskly to either side, then up and down. In alert patients,

### Table 17–2. EYE MOVEMENT FINDINGS IN UNRESPONSIVE PATIENTS

| Patient's Condition | Eyes at Rest | OCR | OVR |
|---|---|---|---|
| Normal, alert | Ahead or volitional, conjugate | Absent | Slow deviation and nystagmus |
| Coma, metabolic | Ahead | Intact horizontal and vertical | Slow deviation to cold, no nystagmus |
| Coma, oculo-motor nerve lesion | Abnormal eye deviated laterally and down | Abnormal eye fails to adduct and elevate | Abnormal eye fails to adduct and elevate |
| Coma, MLF lesion | Ahead or skewed | Adduction fails; vertical OCR normal | Adduction fails; vertical OVR normal |
| Coma, pontine lesion | Ahead or skewed or deviated horizontally away from the lesion | Absent horizontal OCR; vertical may be intact | Absent horizontal OVR; vertical may be intact |
| Coma, mid-brain lesion | Ahead or skewed or vertical deviation | Intact horizontal OCR, vertical absent | Intact horizontal OVR, vertical absent |
| Coma, hemi-sphere lesion | Deviated toward the lesion | Intact | Slow deviation to cold, no nystagmus |

MLF = medial longitudinal fasciculus;
OCR = oculocephalic reflex;
OVR = oculovestibular reflex.

the eyes often go in the direction of the movement. In comatose patients with normal brainstem reflexes, the eyes move conjugately in a direction opposite to that of the brisk movement and then slowly return to the rest position.

### Oculovestibular Reflex Testing

You can also test the *oculovestibular reflexes (OVRs)* of patients whose oculocephalic reflex is unrevealing. Stimuli to test OVRs are stronger than the head turning of OCR. Up to 120 mL of ice water is used to irrigate the tympanic membrane via a small catheter. Make sure that there is no cerumen in the canal, that the tympanic membrane is intact, and that the patient's platelet count is normal. Elevate the patient's head 30° from the horizontal position. A large syringe and butterfly tubing are ideal for this test. Keep a basin underneath the ear to collect the water. You can test the other ear after a 5-minute interval.

In awake patients, cold water results in a slow deviation of the eyes conjugately and horizontally to the irrigated ear (the brainstem's response to the stimulation), followed by a fast-phase nystagmus away from it (a corrective movement originating in the contralateral cortex). Comatose patients with intact brainstem vestibular function and extraocular movement display the slow movement to the irrigated ear, but the nystagmus is absent. Patients with oculomotor nerve lesions have an abnormal eye position at rest; the abnormal eye does not move because of extraocular muscle dysfunction. Patients with medial longitudinal fasciculus lesions have normal vertical movements, but one eye fails to adduct. Patients with lower pontine lesions destroying the vestibular apparatus have no response.

## Localizing Lesions

Different extraocular motor findings are associated with different lesion sites:

- *Dysconjugate eye position at rest,* with the abnormal eye deviated laterally and downward, suggests an oculomotor nerve lesion. In OCR testing, the abnormal eye fails to adduct and elevate normally.
- *Normal vertical eye movements with impaired adduction* on horizontal gaze suggest medial longitudinal fasciculus lesions.
- *A lack of horizontal eye movements* results from low pontine lesions that destroy the sixth nerve nuclei and parapontine reticular formation.
- *Eyes conjugately deviated to one side at rest* reflect either the positive effects of stimulation or a negative response due to a destructive lesion:
  - The eyes of patients with a unilateral destructive hemisphere lesion deviate *toward* the lesion and *away from* the hemiparesis; typically, OCR and OVR can overcome the eye deviation.
  - The eyes of patients with brainstem lesions destroying the parapontine reticular formation deviate *away from* the brainstem lesion and *toward* the hemiparesis; this deviation *cannot* be overcome by OCR or OVR.
- *Normal horizontal gaze with impaired vertical gaze* may be caused by upper midbrain lesions.
  - *Conjugate upward or downward deviation* of the eyes suggests a lesion of midbrain vertical gaze structures.
  - *Dysconjugate vertical deviation* probably represents a pontine or midbrain lesion.

## Recognizing Metabolic Disorders

Patients with metabolic disorders typically have normal extraocular movements, although with deep coma, OCR and OVR may be required to elicit them. Only very advanced metabolic disorders eliminate OCR and OVR responses. **PEARL: Caution is required—antibiotics, benzodiazepines, barbiturates, phenytoin, tricyclics, succinylcholine, and preexisting vestibular dysfunction can impair the OCR and OVR.**

## Motor Exam

Lesions producing coma may damage the corticospinal tract and cause hemiparesis, spasticity, hyperreflexia, and extensor plantar response. However, it may be difficult to detect the hemiparesis of a comatose patient.

Examine the comatose patient for posture, tone, and reflexes. A laterally rotated leg suggests either hemiparesis or a hip or femur fracture. If the patient does not respond to his or her name, painful supraorbital or nailbed pressure can be applied to induce a response. A lack of response yields no information about the status of the motor or sensory systems.

The **"decorticate"** response to a painful stimulus is arm flexion and leg extension, usually reflecting diffuse, severe, supratentorial disease. The "**decerebrate**" response is arm extension and leg extension, usually reflecting a deep hemisphere and upper brainstem lesion. Another response is arm extension and leg flexion, reflecting severe pontine injury. Patients who have only flaccid tone are likely to have dysfunction of the pons and medulla oblongata or diffuse metabolic dysfunction.

Spontaneous movements such as seizures may also occur. Three types of spontaneous movements that suggest metabolic encephalopathy are **asterixis** (jerking of the hands, tongue, or feet), **myoclonus** (shocklike contractions of a muscle or muscle group), and **tremor** (quivering).

## Pitfalls in Coma Evaluation

- The use of drugs or preexisting disease can impair the pupils' reactivity and thus mimic structural coma.
- Drugs or preexisting vestibular disease may cause the absence of extraocular movements, either spontaneous or in response to OCR and OVR testing.
- Drugs and anoxia can eliminate respiratory and motor activity and cause a flat electroencephalogram.

## STRUCTURAL COMA

## Symptoms and Signs

Seek a history of:
- Head trauma (epidural hematoma, subdural hematoma, or brain swelling)
- Progressive neurologic decline (tumor)
- Hypertension, smoking, high cholesterol (stroke)
- Lung or parameningeal infection (brain abscess)
- Fever, seizures, behavioral change, and headache (encephalitis)
- Sudden headache (subarachnoid hemorrhage)

### *Supratentorial Mass Lesions*

Supratentorial masses cause focal neurologic signs and an asymmetrical exam. **Brain herniation** may occur. This is a tissue shift caused by a mass lesion (e.g., tumor, edema); it produces progressive impairment of consciousness and sequential pupillary and motor changes. The change in signs is due to progressive tissue shifts that may result from downward pressure on the thalamus and brainstem (**transtentorial**) or lateral pressure from the medial temporal lobe on the thalamus and upper brainstem (**uncal**) (Table 17–3).

### *Subtentorial Lesions*

Patients with subtentorial lesions demonstrate focal brainstem signs, especially extraocular and cranial nerve disorders, as well as sensorimotor changes. Typically, the focal brainstem signs and the onset of the coma appear at the same time.

## Diagnosis

Computed tomography (CT) and magnetic resonance imaging (MRI) scans can show structural lesions responsible for coma. The MRI scanner must be specially equipped for ventilated patients. A lumbar puncture can help to diagnose enceph-

**Table 17–3. TRANSTENTORIAL AND UNCAL HERNIATION SYNDROMES**

| Herniation Type | Pupils | Eye Movements | Motor Response |
|---|---|---|---|
| Transtentorial | Midposition, no reaction to light | Impaired, dyscon-jugate* | Arm/leg extension or no response |
| Uncal | Pupil ipsi-lateral to lesion dilated and unreactive | Abnormal eye fails to adduct and elevate with OCR and OVR | Hemiplegia ipsilateral to lesion (false localizing sign) |

*As tissue shifts increase and brainstem is increasingly compressed, OCR and OVR progressively deteriorate and ultimately become absent.

alitis or bacterial infection but can accelerate herniation in patients with mass lesions.

## Treatment

Initial general treatment is administered in an emergency fashion, as illustrated in Figure 17–1. The primary problem is treated as soon as possible.

Treatment of herniation should begin no later than the initial detection of pupillary abnormalities. It may begin earlier. Steps include:

1. Partially elevate the head.
2. Intubate with hyperventilation to a $Pco_2$ of 25 mm Hg.
3. Give mannitol (20%) intravenously at a dosage of 1.0 g/kg over 10 minutes with repeated doses of 0.25 g/kg every 4 hours. The goal is 300 mOsm/L serum osmolality.
4. Using normal saline, restrict fluid to two-thirds normal maintenance.
5. If the patient has a tumor or abscess, administer 10 mg of dexamethasone (Decadron) intravenously and then 4 mg by mouth or intravenously every 6 hours along with an $H_2$ blocker; monitor blood sugar.

## DIFFUSE, MULTIFOCAL, OR METABOLIC DISORDERS

### Symptoms and Signs

Patients with diffuse, multifocal, or metabolic disorders usually do not demonstrate early focal signs, but subtle changes of mental status that be-

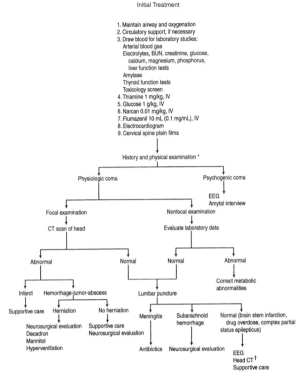

**Figure 17–1.** Algorithm for acute coma management. After initial general emergency treatment of the comatose patient (*top*), management should continue with the history and physical examination in order to determine the primary problem and treat it as soon as possible (*bottom*). BUN = blood urea nitrogen; EEG = electroencephalogram; CT = computed tomography. (Adapted from Furie K and Feldmann E: Disorders of Consciousness. In Feldmann E: Current Diagnosis in Neurology. Mosby-Year Book, St. Louis, 1994, pp 308–312, with permission.)

\* = Includes ice-water calorics, when necessary.

† = If head CT was negative on admission, patient may have brain stem infarction; repeat CT in 24 to 48 hours or obtain MRI.

come progressively more severe. If motor signs are present, they are typically symmetrical and include asterixis, myoclonus, and tremor. Generalized seizures are common. The pupils typically remain reactive. The history may reveal:

- Use or abuse of medication or illicit drugs
- Diabetes
- Alcohol abuse
- Organ failure (coronary artery disease, chronic obstructive pulmonary disease, liver failure, renal failure)
- Thiamine deficiency
- Severe, sudden headache suggesting subarachnoid hemorrhage
- History of seizures suggesting continuous convulsive or nonconvulsive seizure activity or a prolonged postictal state

## Diagnosis

Although CT scanning is often performed emergently, it is often unnecessary with the typical clinical presentation, except to rule out a bilateral and symmetrical subdural hematoma or a co-existing structural process. Lumbar puncture is crucial, especially for elderly patients, even without fever. Lab tests include toxicology screen, tests of organ function ($PO_2$, ammonia, blood urea nitrogen and creatinine, thyroid), glucose, electrolytes, and appropriate cultures.

## Treatment

Antidotes for specific disorders are administered (see Fig. 17–1). These include thiamine, glucose, naloxone, and flumazenil. The primary problem needs specific therapy.

# PSYCHOGENIC COMA

## Symptoms and Signs

Psychogenic coma is not rare. A history of psychiatric disorder and unusual behavior suggests the diagnosis of conversion, catatonia, malingering, or drug overdose. Physical exam may reveal that the lids close actively rather than the slow closure in coma. Pupillary reactions should be normal. During OCR testing, the eyes typically will move with the movement or respond unpredictably. OVR testing, which is uncomfortable, may cause the patient to jump and awaken, or the nystagmus indicates intact hemispheric and brainstem function. The exam is otherwise normal; there are no abnormal motor responses such as decortication or decerebration.

## Diagnosis

Electroencephalography, imaging tests, lumbar puncture, and blood tests are normal. An amobarbital (Amytal, a barbiturate) interview can be performed. Intravenous amobarbital is administered slowly; this drug makes metabolic coma worse but often allows patients with psychogenic coma to awaken slowly. Psychiatric consultation should be obtained.

# OTHER STATES OF IMPAIRED CONSCIOUSNESS

## Brain Death

Brain death is important to identify for prognosis and for humane treatment of the family and patient. The brain is irreversibly damaged, but cardiorespiratory function is intact. Usually there is severe pathology in both of the hemispheres and the brainstem. Specific criteria for the diagnosis differ by institution, but include some combination of the following:

- No evidence of drug use, intoxication, or hypothermia
- Observation for 6 to 24 hours
- No response to painful stimulation above the neck; extensor plantar responses, decerebration, or other responses below the neck may be present
- Absent pupillary light and corneal reflexes, and no response to OVR testing
- No spontaneous respiration on an apnea test (no breathing after apneic oxygenation results in a $PCO_2$ greater than 60 mm Hg)
- Ancillary criteria such as a flat electroencephalogram or no cerebral blood flow

## Persistent Vegetative State

Persistently vegetative patients often emerge from coma with a relatively intact brainstem but diffuse hemisphere damage. They appear wakeful but have no appropriate responses to their environment and no apparent cognitive function. This eyes-open, unresponsive state replaces eyes-closed coma after approximately 2 weeks. The patients' eyes open to voice and sleep-wake cycles, but they do not speak or respond to commands. They may withdraw to pain but do not have any localizing motor responses. Brainstem reflexes are normal.

## Locked-in State

Patients who are in a locked-in state usually have severe brainstem damage with relative sparing of the hemispheres. The damage relatively selectively affects the corticobulbar and corticospinal tracts. Mental status is normal, but only blinking and vertical gaze are spared to allow patient communication. This state is usually caused by basilar artery occlusion or central pontine myelinolysis. It also can occur in severe peripheral disorders such as acute inflammatory demyelinating polyneuropathy.

# *18*
## CHAPTER

# *Status Epilepticus*

Seizures that continue for more than 10–15 minutes or occur in succession without recovery of consciousness are referred to as **status epilepticus** (often known simply as "status"). Although 30 minutes was previously used as an arbitrary cutoff time, we now recognize that a continuous seizure lasting for more than 10 to 15 minutes can have dangerous consequences.

There are two primary forms of status epilepticus: **nonconvulsive** (without tonic [rigid] or clonic [jerking] movements) and **convulsive** (with tonic or clonic movements). Nonconvulsive status includes absence and complex partial status. Convulsive status includes epilepsia partialis continua (focal motor status) and generalized convulsive status. Generalized convulsive status has the greatest mortality and morbidity, but complex partial status also can have serious long-term sequelae.

## NONCONVULSIVE STATUS EPILEPTICUS

### Absence Status

The patient with absence status appears confused or lethargic; the electroencephalogram shows continuous spike-and-slow-wave discharges or intermittent but frequent discharges of this type. This is *not* a medical emergency. Treat with slow intravenous diazepam (0.1 to 0.3 mg/kg), lorazepam (0.04 to 0.08 mg/kg), or valproate.

## Complex Partial Status

The patient appears confused or dazed, and automatisms are often present. Most often, complex partial status is a series of seizures, and the patient remains confused between seizures. It is a relative medical emergency; therapy should be instituted promptly because persistent cognitive impairment can follow. The condition is treated with intravenous diazepam, lorazepam, fosphenytoin, or phenytoin.

## CONVULSIVE STATUS EPILEPTICUS

### Focal Motor Status (Epilepsia Partialis Continua)

The patient has continuous jerking of restricted muscle groups, usually following an acute or subacute lesion (stroke, infection). This is *not* a medical emergency. Often refractory to antiepileptic drugs (AEDs) for several days, the condition is treated with oral medicines listed in Table 18–1 or with intravenous or intramuscular fosphenytoin or intravenous phenytoin.

### Generalized Tonic-Clonic (Convulsive) Status

These patients have continuous convulsions lasting 15 minutes or more, or repetitive convul-

### Table 18–1. TREATMENT OF FOCAL
### MOTOR STATUS*

*Drugs of choice:* carbamazepine, phenytoin

*Alternative choices:* gabapentin, lamotrigine, phenobarbital, primidone, tiagabine, topiramate, valproate

*Drugs are listed in alphabetical order.

sions without return to wakefulness between episodes. **PEARL: Generalized tonic-clonic status is a medical emergency.**

### *Management*

Management consists of:

- History and physical exam (focal onset? post-ictal features such as unilateral weakness [Todd's paralysis]?). Identify treatable causes (e.g., subdural hematoma, infection).
- Lab studies
  - Serum glucose, $Ca^{2+}$, and $Na^+$ before therapy; consider arterial blood gas.
  - Lumbar puncture performed emergently if meningitis is suspected. **PEARL: Low-grade fever is common in generalized tonic-clonic status without infection.** *Pleocytosis* **(white blood cells in cerebrospinal fluid) may result from status.**
  - Computed tomography or magnetic resonance imaging scans when seizures are controlled.

- General treatment
  1. Stabilize vital signs.
  2. Place patient semiprone with head lowered (to prevent the tongue from obstructing the airway and prevent swallowing of secretions).
  3. Place two intravenous lines.
  4. Administer intravenous thiamine (50 to 100 mg) and dextrose.
  5. Follow blood pressure, heart rate, and res-

**Table 18–2. DRUG TREATMENT OF
GENERALIZED TONIC-CLONIC STATUS**

*Intravenous Benzodiazepine*

Use *either* of these two:
- Lorazepam (2 mg/min up to a total dose of 8–10 mg) *or*
- Diazepam (2 mg/min up to 20 mg)

Lorazepam is preferred and is well absorbed intramuscularly. Watch for respiratory depression and hypotension.

*Long-Acting AED*

Use *either* of these two:
- Fosphenytoin (maximum 100–150 mg/min) up to 22 mg/kg (average adult dose is 1200 mg). The major toxicity is hypotension and arrhythmias; closely monitor blood pressure and electrocardiogram for at least 15 minutes after infusion.
- Phenobarbital (25–50 mg/min) up to a total dose of 20 mg/kg. Respiratory depression is the major toxicity and is more common with concurrent benzodiazepine.

piratory status closely during therapy with antiepileptic drugs (AEDs).
- Administration of AEDs. The goal is to control seizures but treatment can be dangerous. Simultaneously administer a short-acting AED (benzodiazepine) and a long-acting AED (fosphenytoin or phenobarbital). The most common protocols appear in Table 18–2.

This protocol is successful in most cases. If not, intubation and a continuous intravenous drip with a benzodiazepine (e.g., midazolam) or a short-acting barbiturate (amobarbital) is required, or general anesthesia.

## *Prognosis*

The prognosis of generalized tonic-clonic status depends on the duration of uncontrolled seizures and the etiology. The greater the structural brain damage (as in hypoxic encephalopathy), the worse the prognosis.

# 19
## CHAPTER

# *Stroke*

A **stroke** is an acute neurologic deficit produced by ischemic or hemorrhagic vascular disease. You will most often see patients with acute stroke in the emergency room (ER). The aggressive pursuit of an accurate diagnosis is important because when the stroke mechanism is known, treatment options and prognosis become much clearer. In nearly three-quarters of ER patients who have an acute neurologic deficit believed to be vascular, the cause is ischemia.

The criteria to determine the mechanism of a stroke include:

- The patient's vascular risk factors
- History of prior transient ischemic attacks (TIAs), which produce symptoms similar to a stroke but typically last only several minutes
- The temporal course of the deficit
- Accompanying symptoms
- The results of the neurologic exam

The diagnosis of stroke requires that history, physical exam, and magnetic resonance imaging (MRI) or computed tomography (CT) exclude a seizure, migraine, tumor, subdural hematoma, or metabolic deficit (hypoglycemia), all of which may mimic a TIA or stroke. Physicians then use clinical features and a head MRI or CT scan to de-

cide upon a presumptive stroke mechanism.
Short-term therapy and supportive care are instituted. An orderly sequence of tests then finalizes
the diagnosis so that long-term therapy can be
started.

CT scanning of the head is the primary method
of imaging strokes. *Hemorrhages* appear as high-
intensity (white) lesions. Intracerebral hemorrhages appear as masses of blood within the brain
parenchyma. If the blood is in a ventricle, cistern,
or sulcus, the diagnosis is subarachnoid hemorrhage. Unlike hemorrhages, *infarctions* are low-
density (dark) lesions that are usually confined to
the territory of a single artery. If there is occlusion
of a large artery or a cardiac embolism, the infarction usually involves cortical and deep tissue.
(If multiple cardioembolic infarcts have occurred,
several arterial territories may be involved.) Infarcts involving small arteries are lesions of less
than 1 cm that are confined to the hemispheric
white matter, thalamus, brainstem, or basal ganglia.

**PEARL: CT and other lab tests do *not* substitute for
clinical evaluation. A CT scan is usually normal during the first 24 hours after ischemic stroke.** MRI has
superb anatomic resolution and may be abnormal
within hours after ischemic stroke, but like CT,
MRI provides only indirect evidence of the stroke
mechanism. For example, stroke due to stenosis
of the internal carotid artery looks similar to
stroke due to cardiac embolism.

Carotid and transcranial ultrasound noninva-
sively examines the extracranial and intracranial
vasculature for occlusive lesions; accuracy is about
90%. Magnetic resonance angiography (MRA) non-
invasively examines the vasculature with similar
accuracy.

Angiography is the gold-standard study of cerebrovascular anatomy. The incidence of complications such as stroke after angiography is less than

1%. Angiography is most commonly performed to image internal carotid disease, extracranially, in carotid endarterectomy candidates. The identification of intracranial disease such as atherosclerosis and dissection may also be extremely important. The angiogram may show unsuspected fibromuscular dysplasia, vasculitis, the vasculopathy of drug abuse, or occlusion of veins. However, the cost and invasiveness of angiography have led to the use of ultrasound and MRA to investigate these patients, with angiography used when the diagnosis remains in doubt. In patients with brain hemorrhage, angiography is still the diagnostic test of choice to reveal the aneurysms and arteriovenous malformations responsible for subarachnoid hemorrhage and, on occasion, intracerebral hemorrhage.

Patients with suspected cardioembolic stroke may require cardiac investigation with echocardiography (transthoracic and transesophageal) and 24-hour Holter monitoring.

Lumbar puncture (LP) is useful for confirming the presence of subarachnoid hemorrhage when a CT scan fails to reveal blood in a patient in whom the diagnosis is suspected. White blood cell abnormalities on LP identify meningeal inflammation in some young patients with unexplained infarction and in other patients in whom the diagnosis of vasculitis is suspected.

## INTRACEREBRAL HEMORRHAGE

Intracerebral hemorrhage originates from small penetrating arteries that branch from major intracranial vessels such as the middle cerebral artery. The arteries eventually weaken and bleed due to wall damage by lipohyalinosis and fibrinoid necrosis in patients with chronic hypertension. The hemorrhages occur in a variety of locations:

- Putamen and internal capsule (40%)
- Frontal, parietal, temporal, or occipital lobe (30%)
- Cerebellum (15%)
- Thalamus (10%)
- Pons (5%)

If the site is atypical or the patient nonhypertensive, consider other etiologies such as amyloid angiopathy, sympathomimetic abuse, aneurysm or arteriovenous malformation, trauma, anticoagulant therapy, or bleeding into a tumor.

The patient usually has elevated blood pressure but not prior warning spells or TIAs. Neurologic symptoms begin suddenly while the patient is active and evolve gradually over minutes to hours. Rebleeding, signified by a sudden, delayed worsening of symptoms, is unusual. Nausea, vomiting, headache, and impaired alertness may occur. The symptoms and signs reflect the site and size of bleeding. Hemorrhages larger than 3 cm in diameter and those close to the midline, which produce brainstem compression, carry a more dire prognosis. CT scan reliably diagnoses virtually all hemorrhages more than 1.5 cm in diameter and misses only small pontine hemorrhages.

Reserve further testing to identify a source of hemorrhage. In nonhypertensives and patients with multiple or atypically located hemorrhages, exclude aneurysm, arteriovenous malformation, and tumor. An MRI is the initial test of choice to screen for underlying lesions. Angiography will be necessary to rule out aneurysm.

Acute treatment must avoid extreme reductions of blood pressure because modest hypotension in such patients can produce global cerebral ischemia. Blood pressure should be reduced only if it is higher than 200/100 mm Hg and then only into the high-normal range. Standard anticonvulsants are used if the patient suffers seizures. For acute and extreme intracranial hypertension, patients are treated with hyperventilation and hyperosmotic agents. Steroid use is not routinely recommended. If a treatable cause of bleeding exists, such as vitamin K deficiency, warfarin therapy, or low platelet count, appropriate replacement therapy may be instituted.

*CONTROVERSY: Surgery for intracerebral hemorrhage is controversial and is usually reserved for large (greater than 3 cm) lobar or cerebellar hemorrhages or deeper hemorrhages with medically uncontrolled intracranial hypertension.*

## SUBARACHNOID HEMORRHAGE

In 85% of patients who have a spontaneous (nontraumatic) subarachnoid hemorrhage, the bleeding comes from a saccular aneurysm. Arteriovenous malformations account for roughly 8%, and the cause of the rest is unknown. Ninety percent of aneurysms are in the anterior half of the circle of Willis.

Aneurysms are usually asymptomatic until they rupture. Rarely, patients suffer short-lived, severe "sentinel" or warning headaches. Rupture occurs while the patient is active and produces sudden, severe headache with or without loss of consciousness. Up to 25% of patients have seizures at onset. After rupture, the patient may be awake and complain of headache. Focal signs such as hemiparesis are unusual. Most patients have impaired consciousness, nuchal rigidity, subhyaloid or preretinal hemorrhages, and fever during the first week. The Hunt and Hess scale (Table 19–1)

**Table 19–1. HUNT AND HESS RATING
OF PATIENTS WITH
SUBARACHNOID HEMORRHAGE**

| Grade | Clinical Presentation |
| --- | --- |
| I | Asymptomatic or slight headache |
| II | Moderate to severe headache, stiff neck, no focal signs other than cranial nerve palsy |
| III | Drowsy, mild focal deficit |
| IV | Stupor, hemiparesis |
| V | Deep coma, decerebration |

grades the clinical severity of subarachnoid hemorrhage. The patient's grade on arrival at the hospital is the best predictor of survival. The mortality of subarachnoid hemorrhage ranges from 5% to 95%, depending on the Hunt and Hess grading. Overall mortality is 50%.

**PEARL: Every patient with severe headache, maximal in intensity at its onset, requires evaluation for subarachnoid hemorrhage.**

Complications are common and serious. Rebleeding is unpredictable but often occurs between days 2 and 19 after initial rupture. About 40% of patients rebleed, of which about 50% die. If an aneurysm is not clipped and the patient survives, the long-term rebleeding rate is 3% per year.

**Vasospasm,** defined angiographically as severe narrowing of intracranial arteries, occurs in approximately 30% of patients. Not all patients with angiographic vasospasm have symptoms, which include headache, ischemia, and raised intracranial pressure. Vasospasm occurs between days 4 and 14 after bleeding and is associated with the presence of thick clot in the subarachnoid space.

CT scan reveals blood in the subarachnoid space of approximately 75% of patients within 48 hours after bleeding. When contrast is given, the aneurysm itself can be seen in up to 50% of cases, depending on the site and size of the aneurysm, the CT scan quality, and whether fine cuts were obtained.

If the CT scan reveals no blood in suspected cases, an LP is performed. If the puncture results are negative, the diagnosis of subarachnoid hemorrhage should be seriously questioned. In true subarachnoid bleeding, lumbar puncture reveals $10^3$ to $10^6$ red blood cells per cubic millimeter. The opening pressure is elevated, and the fluid may be xanthochromic. **Xanthochromia** is a yellowish coloring of the fluid produced by blood breakdown products that appear no earlier than 2 to 4 hours after bleeding. An elevated opening pressure and xanthochromic fluid do not occur with a **traumatic tap,** when blood is released into the fluid at the time of puncture (see Chapter 2). Fluid testing for xanthochromia is performed by spectrophotometric methods, if available, or more simply by spinning the red cells down into a pellet, inspecting the supernatant, and testing it for bilirubin with a dipstick. In a traumatic tap, the red cell count between tubes 1 and 4 may decrease dramatically. This decrease is rare in true subarachnoid hemorrhage. A secondary cerebrospinal fluid leukocytosis with elevated protein may be found 48 hours after true bleeding.

Angiography definitively shows the aneurysm and may also show vasospasm. Four-vessel angiography is required because about 20% of patients harbor multiple aneurysms. A few patients, particularly those with perimesencephalic bleeds, have no aneurysm.

The treatment of subarachnoid hemorrhage depends on the patient's clinical grade. Physicians balance immediate surgery with a conservative "waiting" approach. Waiting increases the risk that rebleeding will occur. Early surgery risks higher operative morbidity and mortality because the brain is acutely swollen and ischemic, and surgery may trigger more severe vasospasm than might have occurred without surgery. One approach to patients in grades I and II is to perform angiography and surgery immediately. Clot is evacuated and the aneurysm is clipped as soon as possible. For patients in grades III to V, whose prognosis is much worse, surgery is postponed until they improve to grades I or II, if they are going to be operated on at all. For these patients, the surgeons wait until the period of high risk for vasospasm has passed. During this period, the patients are usually put at bed rest and given stool softeners, antiepileptic drugs, and sedatives. Docusate (1 to 2 tablets daily) and phenytoin (100 mg po tid) usually suffice. The blood pressure is tightly controlled if elevated.

Nimodipine (60 mg orally every 4 hours) is used to prevent the consequences of vasospasm. If symptomatic vasospasm occurs, the patient is usually treated with intravenous fluid loading and induced hypertension. Some centers use angioplasty or papaverine if vasospasm resists these treatments. Treating vasospasm is less risky if the aneurysm has been clipped.

## LARGE-ARTERY OCCLUSIVE DISEASE

Atherosclerosis of large- and medium-sized arteries causes large-artery occlusive disease. Typical sites include the internal carotid artery, the proximal and intracranial vertebral arteries, and the basilar artery. Symptoms may result from low flow or from the release of microemboli composed of cholesterol, platelets, and fibrin or clotted red blood cells.

Patients typically have coronary disease, hypertension, myocardial infarction, diabetes, or peripheral vascular disease. TIAs in the territory of the diseased artery may have occurred over a period of weeks to months preceding the stroke, but cerebral infarction can occur without prior TIAs. The stroke is either maximal at onset or stepwise in its early course. Headache is not uncommon, and nausea and vomiting occur, especially if the stroke is in the posterior circulation. The location of the lesion is usually cortical and deep, suggesting a lesion larger than that produced by small-artery occlusive disease.

The results of CT scanning are often normal on the day of presentation, but after 24 hours, it reliably reveals a low-density, dark lesion. The stroke is usually in the territory of one artery and is much larger than a lacuna, which might be the result of small-artery occlusive disease. Ultrasound, MRA, and angiography may reveal the location and degree of the atherosclerosis.

Treatment is both general and specific. General therapy includes keeping the patient's head flat, if low flow is the presumptive mechanism of symptoms. In low-flow states, it is crucial to avoid major iatrogenic changes in blood pressure, blood volume, or cardiac output.

Specific therapy is individualized for each patient. Stroke centers experienced with thrombolytic therapy can reduce the severity of acute stroke in highly selected patients by administering intravenous tissue plasminogen activator (t-PA) (0.9 mg/kg) within 3 hours of stroke onset. **PEARL: Thrombolytic therapy can be effective for all forms of ischemic arterial infarction, including both large- and small-artery occlusive disease and cardioembolic stroke.** Only a small minority of patients with stroke currently qualify for this treatment, usually because they arrive too late in the ER. Neurologists experienced with emergent thrombolytic therapy must carefully identify candidates for t-PA. Treatments designed to further reverse the acute effects of ischemia, such as cytoprotective therapy, are under active investigation.

*CONTROVERSY: Many physicians treat patients with ischemic stroke acutely with heparin for 24 to 72 hours, but the benefits of this approach are debated widely. To date, no randomized trial has demonstrated that heparin used acutely for stroke confers benefit.*

Possible long-term treatment includes oral antiplatelet agents such as aspirin (325 mg one to four times daily), ticlopidine (250 mg twice daily), or clopidogrel (75 mg/day); anticoagulation with warfarin (used for severe intracranial stenoses); and surgical removal of a vascular obstruction (endarterectomy). Patients with symptomatic stenoses of internal carotid artery origin greater than 70% benefit from endarterectomy. Patients with asymptomatic carotid stenoses greater than 60% also benefit, but the gain is small.

## SMALL-ARTERY OCCLUSIVE DISEASE

Lipohyalinotic occlusion of small penetrating arteries (less than 200 μm in diameter) that branch from large intracerebral arteries produces small infarcts called **lacunes**. Atherosclerotic disease at the origin of these arteries and embolism are considered less common causes. Occlusion of the arteries produces small, deep infarctions in very circumscribed areas of the brain. The common "lacunar" syndromes are thus restricted and specific:

- **Pure motor hemiparesis:** weakness without sensory, visual, or language deficit
- **Pure sensory stroke:** sensory loss without weakness, visual, or language deficit
- **Clumsy-hand dysarthria:** ataxic hand and slurred speech
- **Ataxic hemiparesis:** unilateral weakness and clumsiness

Small-vessel occlusive disease may produce TIAs before the stroke, but in contrast to large-artery occlusive disease, these TIAs usually occur over a period of days rather than weeks or months. The stroke usually is maximal at onset or has a stepwise progression. Headache is uncommon, and the syndrome is virtually always one of those listed.

The results of CT scanning may be normal or reveal a tiny (less than 1 cm) low-density lesion in the internal capsule, corona radiata, thalamus, or pons. MRI is more sensitive for detecting such small strokes, particularly in the posterior fossa.

Treatment should involve no acute major changes in blood pressure unless the pressure is greater than 200/100 mm Hg. Thrombolytic therapy may be administered acutely to appropriate patients as already described, as may heparin. Chronic therapy includes general supportive care and treatment of the risk factors, especially hypertension, that led to the small-vessel disease. Patients are also treated with aspirin, ticlopidine, or clopidogrel in the same doses as for large-artery occlusive disease.

Patients with similar small strokes downstream from severe carotid disease or in association with atrial fibrillation are often assumed to have suffered stroke due to those conditions and receive therapy directed at those disorders. It is assumed that these patients do not have active small-artery occlusive disease because carotid disease and atrial fibrillation require more specific, aggressive therapy, and their treatment would simultaneously be useful even if active small-artery occlusive disease were actually present.

## CARDIOEMBOLIC STROKE

Cardiac sources of brain embolism include clot in the left ventricle or atrium, valvular vegetation, and tumor particles from a myxoma. These substances usually lodge in medium-sized branching arteries of intracerebral vessels.

Patients typically have a history of coronary disease, atrial fibrillation, rheumatic heart disease, prosthetic valves, recent myocardial infarction, or cancer.

**PEARL: TIAs seldom occur before a cardioembolic stroke, and the stroke is usually maximal at onset.** Headache is not uncommon, and nausea and vomiting may occur if the stroke is in the posterior circulation. The infarct is usually cortical and deep, occupying a territory larger than a lacunar infarction.

As in large-artery occlusive disease, results of the CT scan are often normal on the day of presentation. When abnormal, the stroke may involve multiple vascular territories and suggest a source of clot more proximal than the extracranial carotid or vertebral arteries.

Be careful in using and interpreting ultrasound and MRA in these patients, who have prominent vascular risk factors and may harbor concomitant atherosclerosis. **PEARL: Before ordering tests, decide whether any findings would alter the clinical diagnosis.** Holter monitoring and transthoracic echocardiography can reveal the source of clot. Holter monitoring can diagnose paroxysmal atrial fibrillation. Echocardiography reveals clot in the heart, an area of segmental hypokinesis, an enlarged left atrium, valvular disease such as mitral valve prolapse, or stenotic or regurgitant lesions of the mitral and aortic valves. Transesophageal echo is more sensitive to the presence of sources of embolism such as patent foramen ovale, aortic arch plaque, or left atrial thrombus.

Acute therapy with t-PA may be used in appropriate patients, as may heparin. Chronic treatment with warfarin to prevent recurrent embolization is usually indicated. The primary source of embolism must also be specifically treated. For example, a patient with atrial fibrillation might be treated with digoxin and quinidine; an atrial myxoma or valvular disease might be treated surgically.

## INFARCT OF UNKNOWN CAUSE

By definition, the mechanism of this condition is unclear. The patient demonstrates symptoms and signs attributable to either large-artery occlusive disease or cardioembolic stroke. Patients with infarction of unknown cause have normal angiography, ultrasound, Holter monitoring, and echocardiography. CT scanning reveals a stroke in the territory of a large artery, but normal angiography argues strongly against intrinsic atherosclerosis as the cause of the stroke. Cardioembolic stroke may be suspected, but the source of embolization cannot be detected. These patients should be evaluated for hypercoagulation disorders, such as the antiphospholipid antibody syndrome.

When no disorder is found, one treatment approach is to anticoagulate the patient with warfarin for a short time, such as 3 months. The pa-

## Table 19–2. MAJOR ISCHEMIC STROKE SYNDROMES

| Arterial Territory | Clinical Features* |
| --- | --- |
| Internal carotid artery | Ipsilateral monocular blindness, contralateral weakness of face and arm more than leg, sensory loss, hemianopia, dysarthria, gaze paralysis<br>*Right side:* spatial dyspraxia and left neglect, dysprosody<br>*Left side:* dysphasia |
| Middle cerebral artery | Similar to internal carotid artery, but no ischemia of eye occurs |
| Anterior cerebral artery | Leg weakness more than arm weakness, sensory loss, abulia, urinary incontinence, frontal release signs, gait apraxia |
| Posterior cerebral artery | *Right side:* left hemianopia, hemisensory loss, hemiataxia, prosopagnosia<br>*Left side:* right hemianopia, hemiataxia, transient amnesia, color anomia, alexia without agraphia, hemisensory loss |
| Lenticulostriate artery | Pure motor hemiparesis or ataxia-hemiparesis syndrome |
| Basilar artery/antero-inferior cerebellar artery/superior cerebellar artery | *Complete:* hemiparesis or quadriparesis with sensory loss, ophthalmoplegia, blindness, ataxia, coma<br>*Medial pons:* internuclear ophthalmoplegia, gaze palsy, nystagmus, ataxia, hemiparesis, touch and position sense loss<br>*Lateral pons:* nystagmus, vertigo, facial palsy, gaze palsy, deafness, ataxia, facial numbness, contralateral pain/temperature loss |

| Arterial Territory | Clinical Features* |
|---|---|
| Vertebral artery/postero-inferior cerebellar artery | *Medial medullary:* tongue, arm, and leg paralysis, touch and position sense loss<br>*Lateral medullary:* pain/numb face, ataxia, vertigo, nystagmus, Horner's syndrome, dysphagia, contralateral pain/temperature loss |
| Thalamogeniculate artery | Pure sensory stroke |

*Patients often have partial syndromes exhibiting only some of the features listed here.

tient is then re-evaluated for a source of embolus. If none has appeared, anticoagulation may be replaced with antiplatelet therapy. If a source of embolism is detected, specific therapy is undertaken. Alternatively, these patients may be treated from the start with antiplatelet agents.

## MAJOR STROKE SYNDROMES

Most of the common stroke syndromes may be classified on the basis of the arterial territory involved and the typical associated symptoms and signs (Table 19–2). **PEARL: The identification of an arterial territory does not necessarily imply a particular stroke mechanism.** For example, stroke in the internal carotid artery territory may be produced by atherosclerosis or by cardiac embolism.

# 20

# Brain and Spinal Cord Injury

## TRAUMATIC BRAIN INJURY

Traumatic brain injury is the leading cause of death for Americans under age 35. *Closed head injuries* (no skull injury or only linear fracture) are much more common than *penetrating head injuries,* which have a mortality rate near 50%.

### Pathogenesis

Traumatic brain injuries are dynamic; changes such as swelling may evolve over hours to days. After severe injuries, recovery and improvement may continue for years. Common types of injury include:

- *Focal parenchymal injury:* There is damage (contusion and hemorrhage) to areas underlying the site of injury **(coup),** or on the opposite side **(contrecoup). PEARL: The orbitofrontal,**

frontal polar, and anterior temporal regions ("bumpers and headlights") are involved most often.

- *Acute epidural hematoma:* A temporal or parietal fracture may lacerate the middle meningeal artery or vein. After a lucid interval, the patient develops progressive headache, impaired consciousness, and hemiparesis. **PEARL: Infants and older adults are less prone to developing acute epidural hematoma:** Noncontrast computed tomography (CT) scan demonstrates acute epidural blood with a convex appearance. These hematomas are almost always managed surgically.

- *Acute subdural hematoma:* This hemorrhage may be unilateral or bilateral, often with early and progressive impairment of consciousness. CT scan demonstrates acute subdural blood with a concave appearance, usually over the cerebral convexities. **PEARL: Diagnosis and treatment of acute subdural hematoma within 4 hours of onset is crucial to improve outcome.** Despite surgical evacuation, swelling in the contused underlying parenchyma may cause neurologic deterioration.

- *Chronic subdural hematoma:* A history of trauma may be trivial or lacking. This type of hematoma is often seen in elderly patients taking anticoagulants, and in coagulopathies. Focal signs of axial dysfunction (aphasia, visual field loss, etc.) may be absent. Headache, impaired or fluctuating level of consciousness, and hemiparesis are the most common presenting features.

- *Diffuse axonal injury:* There is severe shearing of axons in the deep white matter. Results of an initial CT scan may be entirely normal, but a later one will reveal obliteration of the gray-white interface.

- *Diffuse microvascular damage with delayed secondary injury to neurons:* This damage includes injury to tissue at the vascular border zone and hippocampus.

## Diagnosis

A history should be obtained from the patient or a witness. **PEARL: A lucid or semilucid interval before a decline in alertness suggests hematoma or expanding contusion, not diffuse axonal injury.** During the medical and neurologic exam, avoid neck manipulation. The **Glasgow Coma Scale (GCS)** assesses eye opening, motor, and verbal responses; scores range from 3 (deep coma) to 15 (awake and responsive) and are correlated with functional outcome (Table 20–1).

Record and follow pupillary responses. Cervical plain films evaluate neck trauma and are recommended before further evaluation. CT is the best imaging study acutely: It identifies significant contusion, hemorrhage, and swelling. CT bone windows detect skull and sinus fractures. Skull films are of negligible value in acute traumatic brain injury.

Lab tests should include complete blood count, electrolytes, glucose level, arterial blood gases, liver and renal function, blood alcohol, toxicology on blood and urine, and coagulation profiles.

## Treatment Guidelines

1. Protect the airway and maintain vital signs; cardiopulmonary resuscitation should be initiated at the injury site, if needed.
2. **PEARL: Immobilize the cervical spine and regard the patient as having an unstable spine until cleared by a lateral cervical spine x-ray.**

### Table 20–1. GLASGOW COMA SCALE

| Parameter | Response | Score |
|---|---|---|
| *Eye Opening* | | |
| | Spontaneously | 4 |
| | To verbal command | 3 |
| | To pain | 2 |
| | No response | 1 |
| *Best Motor Response* | | |
| To verbal command | Obeys | 6 |
| To painful stimulus | Localizes pain | 5 |
| | Flexion (withdrawal) | 4 |
| | Abnormal flexion (decorticate) | 3 |
| | Abnormal extension (decerebrate) | 2 |
| | No response | 1 |
| *Best Verbal Response* | | |
| | Oriented, converses | 5 |
| | Disoriented, converses | 4 |
| | Inappropriate words | 3 |
| | Incomprehensible sounds | 2 |
| | No response | 1 |
| *Total* | | 3–15 |

3. Intubate and hyperventilate comatose patients (GCS score less than 8) to a $PCO_2$ of about 35 mm Hg.
4. Treat shock and systemic hypotension.
5. Avoid overhydration or use of hypotonic fluids.
6. If intracranial pressure increases, sedate with morphine; induce paralysis as needed with pancuronium. Give mannitol 1 g/kg if needed (0.25 g/kg every 4 hours if serum osmolality is less than 310 mOsm/L). Steroids and barbiturate coma have no clear role.
7. Evacuate surgically accessible significant hematomas.

## Outcome after Moderate to Severe Traumatic Brain Injury

Patients surviving traumatic brain injury are often left with significant problems. In addition to focal impairments such as hemiparesis and aphasia, they suffer personality and intellectual changes such as amnesia. Less easily measured deficits in social and vocational functioning are often most disabling. Treatable problems include post-traumatic epilepsy and psychiatric disorders (depression, anxiety, aggression, apathy).

## Minor Head Injury

Although controversial and poorly defined, minor head injury includes both direct head trauma with brief (less than 15 minutes) or no loss of consciousness and indirect trauma such as "whiplash." Both concussive and nonconcussive head injuries may be followed by a constellation of symptoms known as *postconcussive syndrome.* These symptoms are listed in Table 20–2.

The pathophysiology remains uncertain, but both organic and psychogenic factors are involved. Organic factors predominate during the first 2 to 8 weeks, accounting for the stereotypic symptoms such as headache, dizziness, and impaired concentration. These factors contribute to disordered attention and cognition. Psychogenic factors predominate when there are chronic affective symptoms with depression, anxiety, and easy fatigability. Some patients go on to develop chronic migraine or tension-type headache disorders.

Treatment is symptomatic and supportive. Patients should be assured that their physical symptoms will improve with time. Specific complaints should be treated as warranted. Headaches often respond to analgesics (avoid opioids) or antimi-

**Table 20–2. POSTCONCUSSIVE
SYNDROME**

Headache

Blurred vision

Dizziness or unsteadiness

Impaired concentration,
   thinking, and memory

Emotional lability

Noise sensitivity

Fatigue

Irritability

Depression

Anxiety

graine agents; dizziness and vertigo may benefit from vestibular exercises and meclizine (12.5 to 25 mg every 4 to 6 hours). Cognitive impairments resolve gradually. The symptoms of postconcussive syndrome tend to persist even if litigation surrounding the initial head injury is settled.

## SPINAL CORD INJURY

### Clinical Anatomy

The spinal cord extends from the medulla oblongata to the upper border of the second lumbar vertebra. The cord is enclosed at all levels by vertebral bodies with modular components: the vertebral body proper and its pedicles, laminae, facet joints, and foramina through which the spinal nerves pass. The stability of the spinal cord depends on the column of vertebrae, the facet joints, and the anterior and posterior longitudinal ligaments.

On cross section, every level of the spinal cord has universal components. Lower motor neurons (LMNs) arise in the ventral horns; their axons make up the anterior roots. Wasting, weakness, reflex loss, and hypotonia typify LMN lesions. Upper motor neurons (UMNs) occupy the posterolateral and ventromedial white matter and arise in the cerebral cortex. Weakness, spasticity, and hyperreflexia typify UMN lesions. The anterior roots conduct efferent (motor) and autonomic motor impulses; posterior roots conduct all afferent (sensory) impulses. Outside the spinal cord, roots aggregate into major plexuses: the cervical (C1–C4), brachial (C5–T1), and lumbosacral (T12–S3).

Dermatomes (see also Fig. 1–2) are relevant landmarks to localize root and cord lesions:

C5—lateral shoulder
C6—thumb
C7—middle finger
T4—nipples
T8—xiphoid
T10—umbilicus
L2—groin
L5—medial foot
S1, S2, S3—lateral foot and saddle area

For clinical purposes, the major ascending tracts are the spinothalamic and posterior columns. The spinothalamic neurons cross after entry into the spinal cord. The lateral spinothalamic pathway transmits pain and temperature; the ventral spinothalamic pathway transmits crude touch and pressure; and the posterior columns transmit position, vibration, and two-point discrimination. Although spinocerebellar ascending tracts are present and send proprioceptive impulses to the cerebellum, dysfunction in these pathways cannot be recognized clinically in isolation.

Descending tracts include the lateral cortico-spinal tract, which controls limb movements, and the ventral corticospinal tract, which controls neck and trunk movements. Other pathways, such as the rubrospinal, reticulospinal, and tecto-spinal, are not clinically pertinent. Table 20–3 lists the effects of injuries at various spinal levels on motor function and the activities of daily living.

The autonomic nervous system also traverses the spinal cord and is divided into the sympathetic and parasympathetic divisions. The *sympathetic*

**Table 20–3. MOTOR FUNCTION AFTER SPINAL CORD INJURY**

| Spinal Level | Motor Function | Activities of Daily Living |
|:---:|---|---|
| C3 | None | Mechanical ventilation mandatory |
| C4 | Scapular elevators and diaphragm (patient can breathe and shrug shoulders; respiratory reserve low) | Requires motorized wheelchair, mouthsticks, environmental control<br>Requires assistance for all other personal care |
| C5 | Deltoids, partial biceps, some shoulder abduction | Cannot propel wheelchair by self, low respiratory reserve<br>Can perform light grooming and communication; feeds self<br>Requires assistance in bathing, dressing, transfers<br>Can participate in some sports (with adaptive equipment) |

| Spinal Level | Motor Function | Activities of Daily Living |
|---|---|---|
| C6 | Biceps and wrist extensors | Can propel wheel-chair, achieve independence in personal care requiring full body movement, transfers<br>Drives car, participates in sports |
| C7–8 | Shoulder depressors, triceps, wrist flexors, long finger extensors | Grasp weak, but can become totally independent in personal care<br>Brace ambulation and parallel bars<br>Patient does not have strong grip on crutches |
| T1–5 | Hand intrinsics, some intercostals | All activities of daily living are independent, including floor to wheelchair<br>Patient drags legs with crutches; ambulation not functional |
| T6–12 | Intercostals and abdominals | Improved balance, respiration, stamina<br>Long-leg braces and crutches for ambulation |
| L1–3 | Hip flexion and adduction | Ambulates with long-leg braces and forearm crutches<br>Has no sphincter control |
| L4–S2 | Knee flexion | Ambulates with short-leg braces and forearm crutches<br>Has no sphincter control |

division leaves the spinal cord in thoracolumbar segments and is responsible for adrenergic functions: sweating, increasing heart rate, and "fight-or-flight" responses. The *parasympathetic* division leaves the central nervous system (CNS) in cranial and sacral segments and supports cholinergic functions: digestion and elimination. Efferents from the vagus modulate cardiac, pulmonary, and abdominal organ function. Sacral pathways regulate bladder, genitalia, and the distal colon.

## Kinds of Spinal Cord Injury

### *Mechanisms of Trauma*

**Whiplash,** the most common soft-tissue injury of the spine, is an abrupt hyperextension, then hyperflexion of the cervical spine. **PEARL: There is no spinal cord damage in whiplash.** Treatment includes application of a soft collar, heat, traction, and analgesics.

Significant bony injuries to the spine can be divided into hyperflexion-rotation trauma and longitudinal trauma. The first causes fractures and dislocations, most commonly at C5–6 and T12–L1. The stability of the injury is determined by whether the posterior longitudinal ligament is intact. Fracture dislocations generally produce the greatest cord damage. Longitudinal trauma often produces compression fractures, which are more stable. For example, a C1 (Jefferson) fracture may result from a vertically transmitted trauma such as diving and landing on the vertex of the head. Hyperextension trauma to the cord can damage the anterior ligament and most often affects the C4–5 level. A central cord syndrome generally occurs in older individuals with underlying cervical spondylosis. A "hangman's fracture" disrupts the pedicles of C2. Cervical facet joint dislocations are most common at the C5–6 level. Neurologic involvement occurs in 25% of unilateral and 85% of bilateral dislocations.

The neuropathology of spinal cord injury (SCI) is probably due to vascular compression, which results in ischemic-hypoxic damage. **PEARL: Early treatment with high-dose corticosteroids improves outcome from acute SCI, presumably by reducing inflammatory damage.** Treatment with ganglioside growth factors is currently investigational.

### *Classification*

Spinal cord injuries are divided into complete and incomplete injuries. **Complete injury** results in total paralysis and loss of sensation below the lesion. With **incomplete injury,** some sensory-motor function is preserved. Examples of incomplete injury include the central cord syndrome, with motor and sensory loss greatest in upper limbs. A lateral cord injury results in a Brown-Séquard syndrome, with ipsilateral motor and proprioceptive loss, and contralateral loss of pain, temperature sensation, and touch. Incomplete anterior cord injury results in paralysis and loss of pain, temperature sensation, and touch, but proprioception and position sense are preserved. A cauda equina injury is characterized by LMN symptoms (wasting, weakness, reflex loss, and hypotonia) in the legs and sphincter dysfunction.

## Emergency Management

The most important management principle of SCI is maintaining a high index of suspicion. **PEARL: Suspect SCI in all cases of trauma to the face, head, neck, shoulders, or back.** Symptoms suggesting SCI include neck pain or spasm, loss of sensation or mobility, unconsciousness following trauma, and bowel and bladder dysfunction. Associated symptoms of spinal shock (discussed later) include hypotension, bradycardia, and loss of reflexes. Immediate management may require basic cardiorespiratory resuscitation, including nasotracheal intubation or tracheostomy. Proper spinal alignment *must* be maintained, especially during transport to the hospital; a backboard, cervical collar, and rolled blankets may be needed. The immediate neurologic assessment must include a record of the level of consciousness (GCS), sensation, and voluntary motion.

## Diagnosis

Immediate diagnostic studies for the patient with SCI include a careful neurologic exam, with attention to motor, reflex, and sensory levels and autonomic and sphincter function. **PEARL: Plain radiographs of the cervical spine must visualize the C7–T1 region.** Flexion-extension views may be required to assess stability in patients with subluxation. Myelography and CT help to identify subtle lesions and to plan surgery. **Somatosensory evoked potentials** (a test measuring the results of applying a small electical stimulus to large sensory fibers) may offer a prognostic indicator for incomplete injuries.

## Acute Therapy

Surgery is rarely required for acute SCI. Its primary use is for vertebral column stabilization. In incomplete injuries, emergent laminectomy may be indicated to remove a disk, clot, bone, or bullet. Anterior or posterior fusion can increase stability. Harrington rods are used for unstable thoracolumbar fractures. Stability of the spine can be achieved with various external alignment devices, such as a Jewett brace, Knight Taylor brace, Minerva jacket, Philadelphia collar, or halo. Complete immobilization of the cervical spine is attained with cervical traction devices (Crutchfield, Vinke, or Gardner-Wells tongs). Turning frames are useful to prevent decubiti (bedsores).

## Clinical Presentation and Complications

### *Autonomic Manifestations*

**Spinal shock,** a loss of autonomic and motor reflexes below the level of injury, immediately follows a spinal cord injury. The duration of spinal shock is usually 24 hours to 12 weeks after the trauma. Cardiovascular dysregulation with vasodilatation, cardiac slowing, shock, postural hypotension, and edema may be due to the sympathetic disruption. Thermoregulatory changes may impair heat control and sweating; the patient may assume the ambient temperature **(poikilothermy).** Gastrointestinal effects of SCI include stress ulcers and gastrointestinal bleeding. The loss of sphincter control results in incontinence, fecal retention, and hydronephrosis.

Autonomic hyperreflexia often occurs with lesions above T6. This increased autonomic activity can cause flushing, sweating, slowed heart rate, hypertension, convulsions, and cerebral hemorrhage. It can be life-threatening. It is usually caused by a noxious stimulus below the level of injury (for instance, a distended bowel or bladder). **PEARL: Autonomic hyperreflexia is treated by removing the noxious stimulus, such as by clearing a blocked urinary catheter.**

### *Cardiovascular Complications*

Vasomotor shock, caused by sympathetic loss, is the most common life-threatening sequela of

SCI. Features may include hypotension, bradycardia, impaired temperature regulation, cardiac arrhythmias, and impaired sweating. Treatment involves managing the symptoms. Thrombophlebitis and pulmonary embolism are caused by venous stasis, hypercoagulability, and vessel wall damage. Treatment includes use of elastic stockings, daily range-of-motion exercises, early mobilization, proper positioning, deep-breathing exercises, and fluid repletion. Anticoagulant prophylaxis with low-dose heparin should be given. Orthostatic hypotension and edema may respond to the use of abdominal binders, stockings, and a tilting program.

### *Respiratory Complications*

Phrenic nerve damage occurs in patients with lesions at C4 and above. Patients with lesions below C4 will lose intercostal muscle function. Both groups are prone to pneumothorax, respiratory fatigue, and difficulty clearing secretions. Gastric distension interferes with ventilation. Respiratory care consists of frequent turning, deep breathing, percussion and vibration, assistive coughing, postural drainage, and intermittent positive-pressure breathing. Patients with tracheostomy and mechanical ventilation require routine suctioning. Some patients benefit from phrenic nerve stimulation.

### *Nutritional Complications*

Patients with SCI are in a high catabolic state and are prone to poor wound healing and infection. An associated paralytic ileus may prevent oral feeding. Gastritis and stress ulcers should be anticipated and appropriately prevented with antacids, $H_2$-receptor blockade agents, and sucralfate.

## *Urologic Complications*

During the initial phase of spinal shock, most patients have a flaccid bladder. **PEARL: All SCI patients should therefore have an indwelling urinary catheter.** As spinal shock recedes, the patient may be left with a small, hyperreflexic bladder, which may evolve over time into a large, flaccid bladder. Bladder mechanics cannot be reliably correlated with symptoms of incontinence, urgency, or frequency. Beyond routine urinalysis, urine culture, and antibiotic sensitivity, testing may include an intravenous pyelogram, cystourethrogram, cystoscopy, and cystometrics.

Treatments for the "neurogenic bladder" include external, intermittent, and indwelling catheterization. Antibiotics, antispasmodics, and antiseptics may be required.

## *Skin Complications*

Impaired mobility predisposes patients to the formation of decubitus ulcers, osteomyelitis, and sepsis. These typically occur over bony prominences, especially the ischial tuberosities, sacrum, and trochanters. These complications are best prevented by a rigid schedule of position changes. Protective equipment—such as gel pads, sheepskins, and water mattresses—helps. Decubitus care also involves cleansing and drying decubiti, using antiseptics and antibacterials, physical and chemical débridement, and occlusive dressings.

Another problem is that the patient may not sense hazards such as hot water and cigarette burns.

## *Musculoskeletal Complications*

Spasticity is common in chronic SCI and may cause pain and flexor spasms and interfere with perineal hygiene and ambulation. **PEARL: Some patients require a bit of spasticity in order to stand.** Drugs commonly used to manage spasticity include baclofen, tizanidine, clonidine transdermal patch, and clonazepam. Alternative agents are diazepam and dantrolene. Severe cases may require surgical techniques (rhizotomies, myelotomies, and alcohol and phenol blocks). Baclofen can also be infused directly into the cerebrospinal fluid via an implantable pump. Botulinum toxin injections can selectively weaken excessively tight muscles, such as adductors.

Skeletal system changes in SCI include contractures and bone deposits in the soft tissues. These are best prevented and minimized with rigorous range-of-motion exercises. Orthotic devices are useful. Weak shoulders and arms can be supported with a lap board. A resting splint or a leather wrist support treats wrist weakness.

### *Sexual Complications*

The intactness of erection and ejaculation are a function of the extent of the injury. Sympathetic supply to the genitalia derives from T12 to L2 segments; parasympathetic supply comes from S2 to S4. Men with incomplete injury may experience psychogenic erections. Reflexogenic erections can occur spontaneously or due to mechanical stimulus (e.g., bladder distension); these are more common in men with high levels of injury. Ejaculation is often absent or retrograde, but it may occur with mild injury. Fewer than 10% of male patients achieve orgasm, which is more common with incomplete, lower cord injuries. Intracavernosal injections or intraurethral implantation of prostaglandins may induce erections adequate for sexual intercourse. Sildenafil (Viagra) 25 to 100 mg is a useful oral agent. Fertility in men is severely impaired.

In women with SCI, ovulation and menstruation are usually preserved. The extent of vaginal lubrication depends on the level of the lesion. With UMN injuries, reflexogenic lubrication is usually intact, and psychogenic lubrication is impaired; the converse is seen with LMN lesions. Clitoral and vaginal responses follow the lubrication pattern. Pregnancy is often hazardous because the patient may be unaware of labor. Women may be unable to push during delivery, and forceps may be required. Autonomic hyperreflexia may occur with lesions above T6.

## *Psychological Complications*

Patients experiencing SCI undergo extreme psychological distress. Reactions including denial, anger, bargaining, and depression are commonly seen throughout the acute and chronic phases of injury. Patients will require ongoing psychological counseling as well as psychotropic medications; agents such as tricyclic antidepressants, selective serotonin reuptake inhibitors, benzodiazepines, and neuroleptics may be useful in managing the long-term adaptation to physical disability.

# 21
## CHAPTER

# Brain and Spinal Cord Tumors

## GENERAL APPROACH

### Symptoms and Signs

Brain tumors are generally insidious in onset and relentlessly progressive. The commonest symptoms of a brain tumor are new headaches, seizures (partial or secondarily generalized), nausea and vomiting (due to increased intracranial pressure [ICP] or obstructive hydrocephalus), and progressive neurologic deficits. **PEARL: Brain tumors occasionally have a strokelike onset due to intratumor bleeding; the tumors that most commonly hemorrhage include glioblastomas and metastases from lung cancer, melanomas, and choriocarcinomas.**

Rates of tumor progression depend on the prior state of the brain, tumor type, and location. Many patients with brain tumors are known to have primary systemic cancer.

# Diagnosis

Magnetic resonance imaging (MRI) is the best way to diagnose a tumor as well as associated mass effect, edema, ventricular obstruction, or meningeal extension. **PEARL: Compared with computed tomography (CT), MRI can better detect small tumors, low-grade tumors, and tumors in the posterior fossa.** Gadolinium enhancement helps to distinguish tumor from edema.

Surgical resection for biopsy, debulking, or cure finalizes the diagnosis of tumors in the brain or spinal cord. Angiography or magnetic resonance angiography may be required to assess the vascular supply of the tumor or compromise of vital structures before surgery. Embolization of tumors with methyl methacrylate may reduce tumor size and lessen surgical risks. Lumbar puncture can confirm meningeal spread, which is more common for metastatic lesions (lung, breast) than for primary central nervous system (CNS) lymphoma or glioma.

# Treatment

If the clinical and radiographic picture suggests metastases, the primary tumor should be sought and treated. Negative chest and abdominal CT scans are useful in corroborating a primary CNS tumor, because they help exclude a brain metastasis.

Anticonvulsants are usually started after a seizure occurs, not prophylactically. **PEARL: When tumors are cortical or at the subcortical-cortical junction, anticonvulsants should be started prophylactically and continued during the perioperative period.** If no seizure occurs, they can be stopped.

Raised ICP and edema worsen focal signs, causing headache, nausea, vomiting, and impaired consciousness. Raised ICP and obstructive hydrocephalus may develop rapidly, provoking impending or actual herniation; emergency maneuvers outlined in Chapter 17 are used. When raised ICP is more chronic, dexamethasone, a steroid, is beneficial. **PEARL: Although doses of dexamethasone exceeding the standard regimen (10 mg i.v., then 4 mg p.o. or i.v. every 6 hours) are not often useful, occasional patients respond to higher dosages.** Psychosis, agitation, peptic ulceration, opportunistic infections, myopathy, and hypoadrenalism are possible adverse effects. Steroids should be tapered, titrating dose reductions against the clinical response.

Surgery for brain and spinal cord tumors is valuable if metastases are suspected and the source is unknown, if a primary CNS tumor is highly likely, and if radiation or chemotherapy is indicated. Surgery yields a tissue diagnosis, debulks the tumor, and relieves pressure and obstruction. Improved survival and function accrue to patients with known and controlled systemic cancer and a solitary brain metastasis when it is surgically removed. Hydrocephalus may be treated with a shunt. Surgery is hazardous when the tumor invades major arteries and veins or is deep within the CNS (thalamus, brainstem, spinal cord).

Before surgery, radiation therapy should be planned, determining dose, fractions, and ports. Higher-grade malignancies have a better response. Overall dose determines toxicity; in general, less than 6000 cGy given in hyperfractionated doses of 180 to 200 cGy daily minimizes toxicity. Radiation can be given to the whole brain or focally to the tumor. Toxicity may be immediate or delayed; early toxicity (within 48 hours) produces lethargy, cognitive impairments, and worsened focal deficits. Delayed toxicity (6 to 24 months) is caused by coagulation necrosis of vascular endothelium and may mimic recurrent tumor or present as encephalopathy. **PEARL: Diagnosing radiation necrosis is difficult: Positron emission tomography (PET) scans and perfusion-weighted MRI studies may help.** Radiation necrosis may respond to steroids, debulking, or shunt.

Chemotherapy can be given systemically for a primary tumor that has metastasized to the CNS. It is marginally effective for some primary brain tumors.

## SPECIFIC BRAIN TUMORS

### Metastases

Neurologic complications of CNS metastases should be promptly diagnosed and aggressively treated. Lung and breast cancer and melanoma are the most common sources of solid metastases. Although any location for metastases is possible, they frequently occur in arterial watershed territories; half of patients will have multiple lesions. **PEARL: If there is one metastasis and survival chances are good, surgical resection followed by several months of anticonvulsants is valuable.** Anticonvulsants may then be stopped if no seizures occur. Radiation therapy is given to the tumor bed. When lesions are multiple, whole-brain radiation is appropriate; surgery is occasionally used to relieve focal obstruction.

*Meningeal carcinomatosis* occurs with melanoma, breast, lung, prostate, lymphoma, and leukemia sources. Cardinal symptoms are headache, radiculopathies, cranial neuropathies, and cognitive dysfunction. Serial lumbar puncture, removing 30 mL each time, may be required to capture positive cytology. **PEARL: The most consistent cerebrospinal fluid (CSF) finding with meningeal carcino-**

**matosis is abnormally low glucose.** Neuroimaging may reveal meningeal enhancement, hydrocephalus, or solid metastases. Treatment includes intrathecal chemotherapy through an Ommaya reservoir; radiation is focused on solid tumor sites. Prognosis is poor; lymphomas and breast cancers respond best.

## Primary Brain Tumors

*Astrocytomas* are the most common primary brain tumor. They vary in malignancy and in adults are usually located above the tentorium. If the lesion is malignant, less than one-tenth of patients survive beyond 2 years. Treatment is surgical resection with radiation therapy to a limited field. Chemotherapy provides marginal additional survival; patients should be encouraged to enroll in newer protocols. Patients with benign astrocytomas survive longer after surgery, but these tumors often become malignant later.

Brainstem and optic gliomas are usually treated with radiation alone and have a variable prognosis. Biopsy is encouraged when surgically feasible to establish the diagnosis and exclude curable lesions such as abscesses. Cerebellar astrocytoma, the most common childhood tumor, can be cured surgically. Radiation therapy is reserved for recurrence or incomplete resection.

*Meningiomas* are benign tumors and the second most common brain tumor. Women are more commonly affected, and they may be asymptomatic. They typically occur on the convexities of the brain, on the sphenoid wing, near the sella turcica and petrous ridges, but they may occur at any site, even in the ventricles. When accessible, they can be cured surgically, but they may recur if removal is incomplete. **PEARL: Radiation is an option**

**for treating symptomatic meningiomas that are not surgically accessible or totally resected.**

*Pituitary tumors* are characterized by headache, endocrine disturbances, and visual disturbances from chiasmal compression. Invasion of the surrounding cavernous sinus or temporal lobes is unusual. These tumors vary in size and often secrete either prolactin or no hormones. Prolactinomas are characterized by amenorrhea and galactorrhea in women and impaired libido in men. Tumors that secrete corticotropin or growth hormone are uncommon. MRI is more sensitive than CT in diagnosis. Surgery is used for invasive or very large tumors compressing the chiasm, but bromocriptine therapy reduces the size of prolactinomas and some growth hormone–secreting tumors. After tumor removal, lifelong steroid and thyroid replacement is often necessary. Radiation therapy is reserved for tumors that have spread beyond the pituitary fossa.

*Acoustic neuromas* are of Schwann cell origin and are characterized by progressive hearing loss, dysfunction of cranial nerves V and VII, headache, and eventual cerebellar impairment. MRI is the best diagnostic test. They are benign and surgically curable. Hearing loss is inevitable, but facial nerve function usually can be spared.

*Central nervous system lymphomas* (non-Hodgkin's lymphomas) are most common in immunosuppressed patients (e.g., those with acquired immunodeficiency syndrome) but are increasing in incidence among the elderly. Many patients have multiple lesions and meningeal spread is common. Biopsy and lumbar puncture establish the diagnosis. Systemic chemotherapy is indicated. Surgical debulking, corticosteroids, and focused radiation therapy are also used. Intrathecal methotrexate controls meningeal spread. Median survival exceeds 5 years.

*Medulloblastomas* occur between the ages of 2

and 10 years and in young adults. They arise in the cerebellum and cause cerebellar dysfunction and hydrocephalus. Local and meningeal spread may occur. Complete surgical removal is attempted and shunting may relieve hydrocephalus. If tumor has spread, radiation to the entire neuraxis is indicated. Median survival is 10 years. Chemotherapy is often used for recurrence, which carries a poor prognosis.

*Pineal tumors* often manifest as Parinaud's syndrome or hydrocephalus in young men. Typically germinomas, they are treated with surgery and shunting as needed. Residual tumor may be radiated. Lumbar puncture will diagnose meningeal spread; radiation therapy may cure it.

*Craniopharyngiomas* are tumors in the region of the pituitary stalk that compress the visual pathways. Like pituitary tumors, they may produce endocrine dysfunction. Diabetes insipidus and hydrocephalus may occur. Calcification on skull x-rays or CT scans is a diagnostic clue. Surgical resection followed by radiation therapy is the treatment of choice.

*Ependymomas* are usually benign tumors of the fourth and lateral ventricles or the cauda equina. They may appear at any age. They are treated with surgical removal and radiation therapy. Shunting may be needed for hydrocephalus.

## SPINAL TUMORS

Spinal tumors are typically characterized by back pain, radiculopathy, or cord symptoms and signs. Back pain worsened by lying down or by Valsalva's maneuver or back pain associated with motor, sensory, or bladder dysfunction suggests either a spinal tumor or another spinal disorder such as a herniated disk. Spinal tumors may first produce nerve root dysfunction, including shooting pain, followed by spinal cord symptoms and signs such as bilateral limb weakness and numbness, spasticity, extensor plantar responses, and bladder or bowel dysfunction with back pain. The mainstays of diagnosis are plain films, bone scans, and MRI (the imaging modality of choice). Myelography with CT scanning is used when MRI is unavailable.

## Metastases

*Spinal cord metastases* usually involve the vertebral bodies and later spread to the epidural space, where they may compress the roots or spinal cord; sometimes the tumor metastasizes directly to the spinal cord. Extradural metastases most commonly spread from renal, prostate, lung, or breast tumors, or lymphoma or myeloma. Pain is usually the first symptom. **PEARL: Epidural cord compression is a neurologic emergency. Treatment must be started before motor, sensory, or sphincter dysfunction is evident. Back pain in a patient with known cancer should be regarded as epidural cord compression until proved otherwise.** Evaluation involves plain films (looking for pedicle erosion or pathologic fracture), bone scan, and MRI. High-dose dexamethasone, in doses of 25 mg every 6 hours, is started as soon as the diagnosis is suspected and then tapered as definitive therapy with radiation or surgery begins. Metastases may be treated with radiation or chemotherapy if pain is the only symptom. Radiation therapy should encompass both the upper and lower extent of epidural lesions.

A biopsy is justified when no tissue diagnosis is available or no primary tumor has been diagnosed. Some patients with vertebral body tumors secondarily compressing the cord may be treated with anterior vertebral body resection. These patients would not be given radiation therapy and should be in acceptable physical condition for surgery.

**PEARL: The neurologic prognosis is related to the patient's functional status at the time of diagnosis and treatment: Patients walking when treatment is started typically continue to walk, whereas those who are paraplegic rarely regain walking.** Myeloma, breast cancer, and lymphoma are most responsive to treatment.

Because of coagulation necrosis and edema, patients may experience recurrent symptoms and signs of spinal cord compression during radiation therapy, so dexamethasone doses may have to be temporarily increased. Later, some patients develop a progressive, dose-related myelopathy. Residual or recurrent tumor needs to be ruled out. In patients with radionecrosis, imaging typically reveals no tumor, and CSF is normal.

## Primary Tumors

Primary spinal cord tumors may be outside the cord (**extramedullary**) or inside it (**intramedullary**). *Schwannomas* are extramedullary, intradural tumors that produce radicular symptoms and signs, followed by cord compression. They can be cured surgically.

*Meningiomas* in the spinal cord are also extramedullary and intradural, usually affecting the thoracic cord. They often produce radiculoathies. They are benign, slow growing, and more common in women than in men. They can be cured surgically.

*Astrocytomas* infiltrate the cord and are difficult to cure; an associated syrinx (a cavitation in the cord) can be decompressed or shunted. Residual tumor can be radiated.

*Ependymomas* are usually resected for cure.

*Appendixes*

# A

# A Screening Neurologic Examination

| Maneuver | What Is Tested |
|---|---|
| Visual acuity | Cranial nerve II |
| Funduscopic exam | Cranial nerve II |
| Visual fields by confrontation | Cranial nerve II |
| Pupillary light reflexes | Cranial nerves II and III |
| Extraocular movements and convergence | Cranial nerves III, IV, VI |
| Corneal reflex | Cranial nerves V and VII |
| Close eyes | Cranial nerve VII |
| Show teeth, smile, whistle | Cranial nerve VII |
| Weber, Rinne, whisper, watch tick | Cranial nerve VIII |
| Open mouth, say "ah," watch palate | Cranial nerves IX and X |
| Gag reflex | Cranial nerves IX and X |
| Shrug shoulders, turn head | Cranial nerve XI |

| | |
|---|---|
| Stick out tongue | Cranial nerve XII |
| Arms out with eyes closed (drift) | Corticospinal tracts |
| Arms drift downward with eyes closed | Cerebellum, proprioception |
| Fingers show pseudo-athetosis with eyes closed | Proprioception |
| Finger-nose-finger, eyes closed | Cerebellum, proprioception |
| Finger-nose-finger, eyes open | Cerebellum |
| Spread fingers against resistance | Corticospinal tracts |
| Snap fingers, rapid tapping movements | Corticospinal tracts |
| Deep tendon reflexes, jaw jerk | Corticospinal tracts |
| Hoffmann's reflex | Corticospinal tracts |
| Babinski's sign | Corticospinal tracts |
| Heel-knee-shin | Cerebellar system |
| Cotton sensation: face, hands, feet | Spinothalamic tracts |
| Pinprick sensation | Spinothalamic tracts |
| Vibration sensation, 128-Hz tuning fork | Posterior columns |
| Joint position, fingers and toes | Posterior columns |
| Station and posture | Multiple systems |
| Walk, turn, arm swing | Multiple systems |
| Tandem gait (heel-to-toe) | Cerebellar system |
| Deep knee bend | Proximal motor strength |
| Walk on heels | Distal motor strength |
| Walk on toes | Distal motor strength |
| Hop on each foot | Corticospinal tracts, cerebellum, proprioception (multiple systems) |
| Balance on each foot | Multiple systems |

| | |
|---|---|
| Tap soles with heels fixed on floor | Corticospinal tracts |
| Tap heels with ankles dorsiflexed | Cerebellar system |
| Romberg maneuver | Posterior columns |

# B
**APPENDIX**

# *Constellation of Signs by Systems*

### Pyramidal System (UMN)

Weakness, distal greater than proximal
Reduced pendulousness
Spasticity, clasp-knife rigidity, contractures
Retarded performance
Abnormal associated movements
    Arm pronation
    Trunk thigh sign
    Reduced arm swing
    Contralateral movements
Hyperactive reflexes, clonus
Extensor plantar reflexes (Babinski)

### Extrapyramidal System

Tremor
Hyperkinesias
    Chorea
    Athetosis
    Dystonia
    Ballism
Rigidity
    Cogwheel
    Plastic
    Tendon shortening

Postural deformity and instability
Hypomimia
Akinesia
Micrographia

### Lower Motor Neuron (LMN)

Weakness, flaccidity
Fasciculation
Atrophy
Reduced or absent deep tendon reflexes
Trophic changes

### Cerebellar System (Symptoms are ipsilateral to the involved cerebral hemisphere)

Finger-to-nose, heel-knee-shin
Intention tremor
Ataxia
Lack of check
Rebound
Decomposition of movement
Hypotonia
Pendulousness
Macrographia
Dysdiadochokinesis
Deviation on arm extension
Past pointing
Circle walking

### Gaits

Hemiplegic
Paraplegic
Dystonic
Steppage
Waddling
Antalgic
Magnetic
Cerebellar ataxic
Sensory ataxic
Festinating
Astasia-abasia
Dancing
Scissoring
Marche à petits pas

# *Index*

An *f* following a page number indicates a figure; a *t* indicates a table.